Houda Romdhane
Linda Khefacha
Rihem Mezrigui

Autoimmune hemolytic anemias in children

Houda Romdhane
Linda Khefacha
Rihem Mezrigui

Autoimmune hemolytic anemias in children

Mysteries and challenges

ScienciaScripts

Imprint

Any brand names and product names mentioned in this book are subject to trademark, brand or patent protection and are trademarks or registered trademarks of their respective holders. The use of brand names, product names, common names, trade names, product descriptions etc. even without a particular marking in this work is in no way to be construed to mean that such names may be regarded as unrestricted in respect of trademark and brand protection legislation and could thus be used by anyone.

Cover image: www.ingimage.com

This book is a translation from the original published under ISBN 978-620-2-26587-4.

Publisher:
Sciencia Scripts
is a trademark of
Dodo Books Indian Ocean Ltd. and OmniScriptum S.R.L publishing group

120 High Road, East Finchley, London, N2 9ED, United Kingdom
Str. Armeneasca 28/1, office 1, Chisinau MD-2012, Republic of Moldova, Europe
Managing Directors: Ieva Konstantinova, Victoria Ursu
info@omniscriptum.com

Printed at: see last page
ISBN: 978-620-2-71335-1

Table of contents

Introduction

Autoimmune hemolytic anemia (AIHA) is the pathological condition caused by the binding of antibodies (AAs) directed against autoantigens expressed on the surface of red blood cells (RBCs). These antibodies are responsible for the premature destruction of red blood cells, leading to more or less severe anemia [1].

AHAI is known as a relatively rare cause of anemia, but represents the most common form of acquired extracorporeal hemolysis in children [2].

Mechanisms of hemolysis differ for the different types of AHAI, depending on the class, sub-class and ability of the autoantibody (AAC) to activate complement [3].

The diagnosis of AHAI requires not only the demonstration of anaemia of varying degrees, secondary to the shortening of red cell life (haemolysis), but also the presence of AAC [1] .

The clinical expression of this pathology makes it a particularly heterogeneous entity, ranging from fully compensated forms with progressive development to those with rapid onset and a life-threatening prognosis [4].

Its history is intertwined with that of paroxysmal cold hemoglobinuria (PCH). Indeed, the first description of an autoimmune disease mediated by AACs was made by Donath and Landsteiner in 1904, and these AACs were responsible for cold paroxysmal hemoglobinuria [3].

In 1938, the existence of acquired hemolytic anemias involving an AAC was definitively established.

An important diagnostic advance, essential to the elucidation of the pathophysiology of AHAI, occurred in 1945 with the description of the antiglobulin test by Coombs, Mourant, and Race. Since then, in the 2 decades since the 1950s, major advances have been made in diagnostic tools, etiological hypotheses, pathogenesis and new therapeutic procedures for AHAI [3].

In recent years, new studies have led to a clear improvement in scientific knowledge of this pathology, particularly in terms of immunohematology and clinical aspects. Numerous pathological associations have been reported, but a cause-and-effect relationship has rarely been established. Therapeutic modalities, a major challenge, remain largely dependent on etiological approaches that are often difficult to establish.

In this work based on a retrospective study of 17 cases of AHAI, diagnosed in the pediatric department of the Farhat Hached University Hospital in Sousse, we aimed to:

- ❖ Study the epidemiological profile of AHAI in children
- ❖ Study the clinico-biological and etiological profile of this pathology
- ❖ Present current therapeutic modalities
- ❖ Analyze how the disease evolves.

1.   Bibliographic reminder

1.1. Etiopathology

Autoimmune diseases are the result of diverse pathophysiological mechanisms involving the interplay of genetic and environmental factors. Despite the accumulation of numerous, sometimes highly suggestive observational facts, the proposed patterns of AAC onset still remain relatively hypothetical [5,6].

Several factors involved in autoimmunization have been reported.

1.1.1. Genetic predisposition

Genetic predisposition is an essential factor in the development of autoimmune diseases, including AHAI. Genetic studies carried out in animal models of autoimmune diseases have shown that there are at least 25 genes that may contribute to a particular susceptibility to autoimmune diseases. These genes mainly code for major histocompatibility complex (MHC) class I and class II proteins, cytokines, cytokine receptors and proteins involved in immune response regulation and apoptosis. This is supported by the existence of familial forms in some AHAI patients [5-7].

1.1.2. Immune system dysregulation

Numerous observations, particularly in prolonged or chronic AHAI, support the hypothesis of a central immune dysfunction, with multiple determinants, at the origin of the appearance of AAC without the active intervention of RBCs. The frequent changes in the nature and specificity of AAC during the course of the disease are clues that practically eliminate the direct or indirect responsibility of RBCs as the inducing agent of autoimmunization [6].

1.1.2.1. Suppressor T-cell deficiency

The loss of T lymphocyte suppressive functions towards B lymphocytes is a working hypothesis that has already been documented in humans in the lupus syndrome, which is very similar to idiopathic AHAI [6].

In humans, very few data are available on the potential role of regulatory T cells in AHAI. Studies by Hall et al. have shown that in the peripheral blood of AHAI patients, there are Rhesus system (RH) autoantigen-specific regulatory T cells capable of inhibiting the Th1 effector T cell immune response in vitro via an interleukin 10 (IL-10)-dependent mechanism [8]. More recently, Ahmad et al. showed a significant decrease in the level of regulatory T lymphocytes (4.63% vs. 9.76%) in AHAI patients compared with healthy donors [9].

1.1.2.2. Polyclonal activation of B lymphocytes

Polyclonal activation of both B and T cells is likely to play a role in the induction of AHAI.

In patients with "hot" AHAI compared with healthy subjects, there is an imbalance in the th1/th2 balance of CD4+ *helper* T cells. An increased proportion of Th2 cells and expression of both interleukin 4 (IL-4) and IL-10, and reduced expression of interferon-y and IL-12 were noted. This "Th2 cell profile" favours the induction and proliferation of autoreactive B cells [1, 9, 10].

1.1.2.3. Lack of Fas-dependent apoptosis

A defect in lymphocyte apoptosis secondary to a mutation in the gene encoding the Fas death receptor can induce lymphoproliferative syndrome with autoimmunity (LPSAS) in humans [11]. The most frequent autoimmune manifestations in this nosological context are mainly hematological: hemolytic anemia, thrombocytopenia, neutropenia. This syndrome is characterized by :

- Non-malignant lymphoproliferative syndrome (splenomegaly, adenopathy)
- Autoimmune manifestations.
- An expansion of a rare but normal population of circulating or tissue lymphocytes (double-negative T lymphocytes).
- In vitro resistance to apoptosis in cultured T and B lymphocytes.

Various constitutional heterozygous mutations of the Fas gene have been identified in children with SLPA.

The interaction of the Fas receptor with its ligand Fas L (for Fas ligand) induces apoptosis or programmed cell death. Fas (CD95) is a type I transmembrane glycoprotein belonging to the TNF (*Tumor Necrosis Factor*) receptor superfamily. It plays a key role in T and B lymphocyte homeostasis. The important role of this apoptotic pathway has been demonstrated in vivo in mouse models [7].

1.1.3. Alteration of the erythrocyte membrane: role of the autoantigen

Some AHAIs are characterized by a significant weakening of the expression of certain erythrocyte antigens. Restoration of normal antigen expression is followed by disappearance of the AACs.

In animals, AACs can be produced following injection of autologous RBCs altered by heating or formalin. Anti-I cold agglutinins have been produced in rabbits following injection of human RBCs previously incubated in the presence of *Mycoplasma pneumoniae*.

The appearance, under the effect of certain bacterial enzymes, of T or Tn crypto-antigens is a particular situation in which anti-T or anti-Tn antibodies, normally present in human plasma, can react with autologous RBCs thus modified and lead to their premature destruction [6].

In children, significant hyper-expression of CD99 (GR membrane markers) has been demonstrated. Over-expression of this adhesion molecule may be involved in the enhanced leukocyte-RG-platelet contact that precedes the destruction of RBCs and platelets [12].

1.1.4. Normal immune response and cross-reactivity

The hypothesis of a certain structural kinship between antigens in the RBC membrane and those of external aggressors is also one of the mechanisms by which anti-erythrocyte AACs are induced.

Immunization of rabbits with *Lysteria monocytogenes* causes the transient appearance of anti-erythrocyte cold agglutinins, which in vitro recognize the immunizing organism. Similarly, in I-negative mice, infection with *Mycoplasma pneumoniae* produces anti-I cold agglutinins. On the other hand, anti-I associated with *Mycoplasma pneumoniae* infection can be inhibited by a lipo-polysaccharide extracted from the germ. It has also been shown that biphasic hemolysin can be inhibited by both globoside P and the closely related *Forssmann* glycolipid [6].

1.2. Pathophysiology

Multiple parameters are involved in the destruction of RBCs in vivo. Some relate to the antigen-antibody pair (Ag-AC), others to the systemic environment, such as the functioning of the complementary system or the purification capacity of the reticuloendothelial system. The multiplicity of these parameters easily explains why not all AACs are hemolyzers, and why the equation AAC = AHAI is not too simplistic [6].

1.2.1. Complement-dependent hemolysis by activation of C1 up to C9

In "cold" AHAI, sensitization of RBCs to the action of complement can lead to their destruction. This is due to activation of the classical complement pathway, leading to the formation of the membrane attack complex (C5, C6, C7, C8 and C9), resulting in cell lysis and release of hematocyte constituents (mainly hemoglobin) into the bloodstream, with hemoglobinemia, hemoglobinuria and a fall in haptoglobin[13, 14].

Intravascular hemolysis is usually an acute event. The anti-erythrocyte AACs responsible for this hemolysis are complement-fixing immunoglobulins (Ig), which are highly hemolyzing in vitro and in vivo. These are biphasic Donath Landsteiner hemolysins (HBDLs) ("cold" IgGs) or certain "cold" IgMs, as well as the very rare "hot" IgMs responsible for often very severe intravascular hemolysis. Cold agglutinin disease (CAD) and HPF are two common examples of such hemolysis. However, other tests suggest that the major mechanism of hemolysis in CFD is hepatic sequestration of sensitized RBCs by C3b fractions of complement [6, 15, 16].

Destruction of red blood cells in the circulation is a relatively rare occurrence. Regulatory complement proteins can inhibit activation of the complement cascade (C5 to C9), in which case hemolysis of complement-sensitized RBCs does not occur [17].

1.2.2. Complement-dependent erythrophagocytosis

Activation of complement by the alternative pathway can lead to recognition of C3b, expressed on the GR surface by the C3b receptor expressed by various cells, including macrophages. The RBC can then be captured and phagocytosed. This erythrophagocytosis mechanism takes place mainly in the liver, involving Küpfer cells and resulting in the clinical picture of extravascular hemolysis. The AACs involved are most often complement-fixing IgG or IgM [13, 16].

Intrahepatic conversion of C3b is responsible for the deposition of C3d on surviving erythrocytes, which are released into the systemic circulation (Figure 1). The C3d fraction is thus the indicator of the sensitization of RBCs to the action of complement. It is this molecule that is recognized by the anti-complement antiglobulins used in the direct Coombs test (DCT). The formation of C3d on the surface of RBCs gives rise to the following phenomena:

> The deformability of RBCs returns to normal, thereby eliminating one of the factors that favoured phagocytosis, namely their acquired rigidity.

> The inability of RBCs to bind other C3 molecules, which removes them from the lytic action of the ever-present AAC [6, 13, 16].

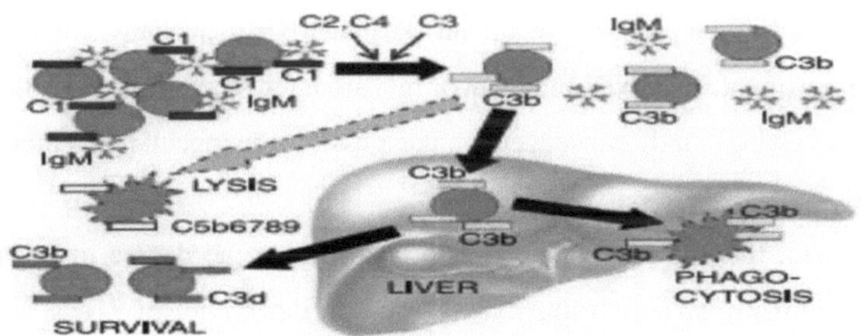

Figure 1: Complement-dependent erythrophagocytosis by liver Küpfer cells in "cold" AHAI[16].

1.2.3. IgG-dependent erythrophagocytosis

In the case of "hot" AACs, as Ig is attached to the surface of RBCs by its Fab fragments, its Fc fragments can be recognized by the receptor for the Fc fragment of IgG, particularly the IGg3 and IgG1 subclasses expressed by various cells including macrophages, leading to phagocytosis of RBCs. This explains the hemolytic role of IgG3 and, to a lesser extent, IgG1, while IgG2 and IgG4 AACs have almost no hemolytic effect [18].

Most of the RBC sequestration phenomena in "hot" AHAI occur in the spleen, expressing a picture of extravascular hemolysis, whereas hepatic RBC trapping occurs for RBCs sensitized by large quantities of IgG or when complement fractions are present on their surface [1, 18].

Erythrophagocytosis may be partial, with the unphagocytosed hematite fragment taking on the appearance of a spherocyte, which in turn is sequestered and phagocytosed in the spleen. Spherocytosis is frequently diagnosed in AHAI. The degree of spherocytosis is proportional to the severity of hemolysis. In principle, the mechanism of hemolysis influences the efficacy of the proposed treatment, particularly splenectomy. Receptors for complement and the Fc fragment of IgG are interesting approaches to the pathophysiology and, consequently, the possible therapeutic potential of AHAI.

At present, there is no reliable test to characterize the degree of in vivo responsibility of an anti-erythrocyte AAC in the destruction of RBCs, as the occurrence of hemolysis depends on multiple factors:

- Quantity of CA fixed: specificity, temperature
- Fixed top-up quantity
- Number of receivers for Fc, for C3b
- AAC affinity
- Type of IgG fixed (IgG1, IgG3) [13, 15, 17].

1.2.3. Antibody-dependent cytotoxicity

ADDC *(antibody-dependent cell cytotoxicity)* may also be another way in which "killer" lymphocytes, like NK *(Natural Killer)* cells, destroy red blood cells. These cells can destroy red blood cells coated with IgG-type antibodies (AC), for the Fc portion of which they have receptors, even in the absence of complement. This mechanism does not require large quantities of ACs, but the integrity of their Fc fragment [6, 9].

1.2.4. Special case of IgA AHAI

The mechanism of hemolysis in IgA AHAI is poorly understood. Booth et al. had shown that allo-IgA did not activate complement, but later Sokol et al. detected complement fractions attached to the erythrocyte membrane, apparently activating the alternative pathway. Hemolysis can also be mediated by monocytes expressing specific receptors for the Fc fragment of IgA. The antigenic target, band 3 protein, has already been reported in young children. This protein is massively present on the surface of RBCs [20].

1.2.5. Special case of drug-induced AHAI (AHAIM)

The mechanisms generally differ from one drug to another, but can be multiple for the same molecule. Three mechanisms are usually proposed:

> ➤ The hapten mechanism, in which CAs react with the single drug adsorbed to the RBC membrane. CAs are then said to be drug-dependent, and their in vitro detection requires the presence of the molecule. Here, identification of the CA in patient plasma requires the latter to be brought into contact with a solution of RBCs previously sensitized by incubation with the incriminating molecule. The main drugs inducing this mechanism are penicillin and cephalosporins.

> ➤ The immune-complex mechanism, in which the ACs bind to part of the drug and to the GR membrane protein. These ACs are also known as drug-dependent, but their detection requires plasma to be brought

into contact with a solution of the free drug and non-sensitized RBCs. The molecules concerned are mainly cephalosporins and piperacillin.

> The autoimmune mechanism, where the CAs correspond to AACs whose main target is a GR membrane protein. In this case, the CAs are drug-independent and do not require the presence of the molecule to be detected. These AHAIM with drug-independent CAs cannot be differentiated from true AHAI on the serological level. Only the disappearance of the hemolytic anemia, generally one to 2 weeks after discontinuation of the drug, or the remote negativation of the CDT, can rule out an iatrogenic origin. The drugs responsible for this mechanism are mainly fludarabine and interferons, as well as alpha-methyldopa; the latter is currently no longer used [21].

1.3. AHAI classifications

AHAI is an extremely heterogeneous and polymorphous group of disorders. One reflection of this polymorphism is the multiplicity of classifications proposed on the basis of clinical, serological and etiological data [6].

1.3.1. Immunological classification

The classification of AHAI depends essentially on immunochemical characteristics, the isotype of the AAC involved and the optimum temperature for binding the AAC to the erythrocyte antigen in vivo. A distinction is thus made between "hot", "cold" and "mixed" AHAIs. This distinction is of both clinical and biological interest, since each of these AHAI varieties has its own clinical picture and treatment [10, 15, 22].

1.3.1.1. Hot" AHAI

These are the most common AHAI, accounting for 60-80% of all AHAI in adults, and around 90% of AHAI in children. AACs are described as hot when they exert their maximum hemolytic activity at temperatures (thermal optimum) of between 35 T and 40° C. They are predominantly IgG. IgG1 is much more common than IgG2, IgG3 and IgG4. The erythrocyte coating consists of :

- IgG in 20 to 60% of cases
- IgG + C3d in 25% to 65% of cases

- C3d alone in 7% to 15% of cases [1, 17].

These AACs can recognize certain specificities. These are usually high-frequency RH system antigens, rather than simple antigens (anti-e, anti-D). GR membrane glycoproteins and phospholipids have also been reported as AAC targets. Hemolysis is intra-tissular and predominantly splenic [10, 22-24].

1.3.1.2. Cold" or Cryopathic AHAI

> AHAI with cold agglutinins

Cold AHAIs are encountered in 15% of cases. These AHAIs are also known as "cold agglutinins" and, by binding to the membrane antigens against which they are directed, are capable of spontaneously inducing agglutination of red blood cells at low temperatures, optimally at +4 T in a saline environment, which has earned them the name "complete CA". This phenomenon is reversible after reheating. They are predominantly IgM and sometimes IgG, always coated with C3d. TCD is also positive, but with complement-recognizing human antiglobulin (complement alone or IgM-complement).

The thermal optimum for cold AAC is +4 T, but the thermal amplitude is variable and can be as high as 37T. The latter must be determined at +4, +22 and 37 T, and has clinical significance. In assessing the pathological nature of a cold agglutinin, not only the titre but also the thermal amplitude must be taken into account. Thus, if agglutination persists at 37T, cold agglutinin is often responsible for hemolysis even at low titre [13, 15].

The target antigenic structures of AACs are "public" antigens: I or i antigens (I in the majority of cases). Pr specificity has also been reported [23-25]. Among cold agglutinin AHAIs, a distinction is made between acute, post-infectious forms and chronic forms known as MAFs, which account for 10-20% of AHAIs in adults and are exceptional in children [26].

Cold agglutinins cause hepatic red cell lysis via complement activation [17, 22].

➢ Biphasic or Donath Landsteiner AHAI

HPF is due to a cold AAC that binds at low temperatures ($< 30°$ C) but only activates complement at high temperatures ($37°$ C), hence the term HBDL. This form is characterized by intravascular hemolysis with hemoglobinuria. In the past, it was suggestive of syphilitic infections. However, it now seems to be the preserve of infantile forms linked to viral infections, not uncommon in children under 16. AAC with biphasic activity is directed against the P antigen with a negative or positive TCD to C3d or weakly positive to IgG. This form of hemolytic anemia (HA) tends to heal spontaneously, sometimes with the help of appropriate transfusion support [13, 15, 23].

1.3.1.3. Special cases

➢ Mixed AHAI

Mixed" AHAIs: result from the simultaneous presence of "hot" IgG-type AACs and "cold" IgM-type AACs. They are most often severe and account for around 8% of AHAI cases. A good response to treatment has been described [17, 14, 23].

➢ AHAI with IgA-type AAC

Among "hot" AHAIs, the presence of anti-GR IgA is particularly exceptional and can lead to fulminant hemolysis [15, 20].

➢ IgA cold agglutinins

They do not activate complement and are not responsible for hemolysis, but only for peripheral cutaneous manifestations triggered by cold [10].

➢ Hot" AHAI with IgM-type AAC

The most dreaded variety, fortunately very rare, is "hot" IgM AHAI. IgM-type CAA has a wide temperature range and agglutinates red blood cells at 37° C. This AC binds complement. Complement activation may be complete up to C9, or stop at C3 due to inactivation processes. TCD is thought to be complement-positive [10, 14, 27].

1.3.2. Evolutionary classification

1.3.2.1. AHAI aigues

Acute forms evolve over a period of less than three months, occurring mainly in young children, more rarely in adolescents and adults. Onset is rapid or abrupt, with hemolysis that is usually intense and often intravascular. In certain circumstances, the hemolytic crisis may follow or coincide with a clinically characterized viral or bacterial attack (rhinopharyngitis, atypical pneumonitis, chickenpox, measles, influenza), or with an undocumented febrile pathology and various vaccinations [6, 12].

1.3.2.2. Chronic AHAI

The absence of remission within three months of onset, or subsequent recurrence, defines the transition to chronicity. Chronic AHAI occurs at any age, but more frequently in adults. The onset may be abrupt, but the anemia is often progressive or insidious in onset, sometimes being discovered only by chance during a laboratory examination [6, 12, 28].

1.3.3. Etiological classification

Depending on the context in which AHAI occurs, a distinction is made between :

- Idiopathic forms, where AHAI is not associated with any other pathology and therefore appears as a primary disease.
- Secondary forms triggered by an etiological agent or forms associated with an underlying disease.

Thus, AHAI can be considered secondary when:

- The conjunction of anemia and underlying disease occurs more frequently than can be represented by chance alone.
- Correction of associated disorders reverses AHAI.
- Anemia and associated disease are linked by evidence of immunological aberration [15, 17].

According to the largest series in the literature, around 45% of AHAIs are considered to be "secondary" or associated with an underlying disease, around 15% are considered to be primary or "idiopathic", and 40% are considered to be attributable to drug intake [29].

Primary "hot" AHAI accounts for around 50% of "hot" AHAI cases. It appears clinically isolated or, at most, associated with thrombocytopenia of variable course, with or without purpura, giving rise to the classic Evans syndrome (ES).

In the other half of cases, known as symptomatic or secondary, AHAI is associated with other complex clinical and biological diseases or disorders, such as haematological malignancies, systemic diseases, lupus, Biermer's anaemia, liver cirrhosis, ulcerative colitis, immune deficiencies and so on. Chronic lymphocytic leukemia and lymphoma account for around half of AHAI with secondary hot AAC [6, 17].

According to some authors, HAIs associated with infections predominate in children. According to others, most cases of AHAI are primary.

Some reports suggest that, in childhood, secondary forms are more frequent than idiopathic forms, and viral and bacterial agents are frequently the only triggering factor. Indeed, AHAI associated with viral infection or secondary to vaccination is much more frequently described in children than in adults [30, 31].

In adults, primary AHAI accounts for around 60% of cases. In paediatric series, the proportion of patients with primary AHAI varies from 7% to 64%, and "hot" AHAI accounts for around 60% of cases.

Some series report that primary AHAI is more frequent, while others show that secondary forms are more common in the paediatric population.

It is important to emphasize that primary AHAI can often follow a viral-like syndrome and precede the onset of another immunological disease for years, in most cases SE [2,32].

2. Materials and methods

2.1. Patients

➢ Patient origin and data collection :

This is a retrospective study, carried out at the Sousse regional blood transfusion center (CRTS), targeting patients in the pediatrics department of the EPS Farhat Hached with a positive TCD.

In the period from 2004 to 2014, around 5993 CDTs were performed for the pediatric department.

Patients with a positive TCD were searched using the "recipient search" module of MEDINFO's Hematos IIG software.

A data sheet has been designed to gather epidemiological, clinical, biological, immuno-hematological, etiological, transfusion, therapeutic and evolutionary data relating to patients. These data were extracted from CRTS transfusion files and patients' clinical records.

➢ Inclusion criteria:

The patients included in this study were all under 16 years of age at the time of diagnosis. AHAI was defined as a hemoglobin (Hb) level below 11 g/dl associated with clinico-biological signs of hemolysis and the demonstration of anti-erythrocyte ACs by TCD. Polytransfused patients with an inherited hemoglobin abnormality associated with AHAI, namely beta thalassemia and sickle cell disease, were not excluded from the study.

All patients who did not meet the inclusion criteria and for whom the available data were deemed insufficient (lost or incomplete clinical records, positive DBT without context, etc.) were excluded from the study from the outset.

2.2. Methods

2.2.1. Epidemiological study

Data collected from patients' medical records included: current age, age at diagnosis, gender and governorate of origin.

2.2.2. Clinical study

We looked for the following in our patients:
- Reason for initial consultation
- The presence of a family history, in particular the notion of parental consanguinity
- Personal history
- The main clinical manifestations of the disease
- Clinical signs revealing pathology associated with AHAI

2.2.3. Biological study

When faced with a clinical diagnosis suggestive of hemolytic anemia, laboratory tests confirming the hemolytic nature of the anemia (LDH (Lactate dehydrogenase), unconjugated bilirubin, haptoglobin) and tests confirming the immunological nature of the hemolysis are performed. These included:

2.2.3.1.   Direct Coombs test

Described by Coombs in 1945, the Coombs Test is a semi-quantitative method for the agglutination of red blood cells, revealing the presence of ACs directed against RBCs, whether bound to the erythrocyte surface (TCD) or circulating (Indirect Coombs Test (ICT)) [13,14, 22].
- Principle and limitations of TCD

The principle of TCD is to use ACs directed against the Fc fragment of human Ig (obtained by immunization of rabbits). In this way, and only if IgG is bound by its Fab fragment to the surface of the RBCs tested, rabbit antiglobulins cause agglutination of these RBCs. This technique also makes it possible (by performing the test with rabbit ACs directed against complement) to detect any complement attached to the surface of the RBCs to be tested. The test is positive if agglutination of the RBCs occurs [13].

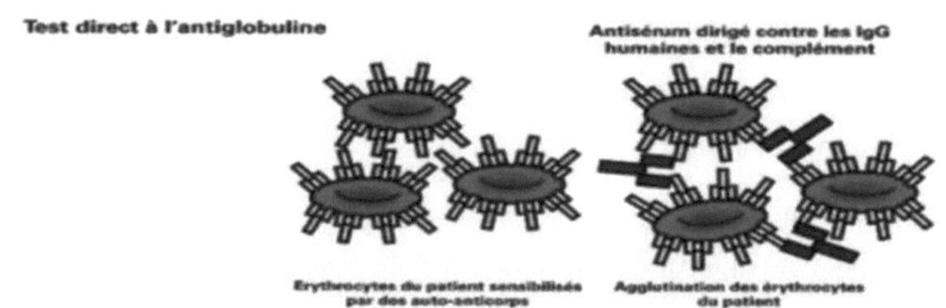

Figure 2: Principle of the direct Coombs test [15].

The test is performed first with broad-spectrum antiglobulin (polyvalent human Ig), which contains ACs directed against human Ig and complement proteins. When agglutination is noted, anti-IgG and/or anti-C3d monospecific Ig is used. In some cases, anti-IgM or anti-IgA monospecific Ig may also be used.

Given the excellent sensitivity of the direct antiglobulin test with current techniques, its negativity virtually eliminates the diagnosis of HAI. However, in the absence of an alternative diagnosis to explain HA, a negative TCD must be supplemented by a TCD using anti-IgA and/or anti-IgM globulin and by elution. In theory, however, in a tiny minority of cases, genuine AHAI with negative TCD cannot be completely ruled out.

According to the literature, TCD-negative AHAI is frequently encountered, corresponding to 5-10% of cases of this pathology, and depends in part on the activity of the Coombs reagent used for the test [20, 22, 27, 33].

There are three main reasons for this negativity in some cases of "hot" AHAI:

- ■ The threshold for sensitization of RBCs by IgG is lower than that for detection by the Coombs reagent.
- ■ Low-affinity IgG is eluted from red blood cells by preoperative washes not performed at +4 T or in low-ionic-strength media. AHAI with low-affinity IgG may be associated with severe hemolysis.
- ■ Red blood cells are sensitized only by low-molecular-weight IgA or monomeric IgM, which do not bind complement, so other AACs are not detectable by the commercial Coombs reagent, which contains anti-IgG and anti-C3d.

Most commercial Coombs reagents have a sensitivity that exceeds the threshold for sensitization of RBCs by IgG capable of inducing immune hemolysis. This threshold is not precise and varies from reagent to reagent. Its lower limit of sensitivity varies from 150 to 500 IgG molecules per RBC, whereas a sensitization level below 150 IgG can induce hemolysis [34]. Previously performed in tubes, TCD on gel micro-columns has better sensitivity and specificity (98.4% to 100% and 83% to 95.2% respectively in recent studies). This solid-phase technique is currently widely used [13, 27].

One of the major advantages of the TCD solid-phase gel filtration technique is that it enables red blood cells to be studied without prior washing, which is known to result in the elution of certain fixed ACs: Antiglobulins (antiserum) and erythrocytes are first incubated in a reaction chamber, then the micro-tubes are centrifuged. If agglutination occurs, the agglutinate is retained on passage through the gel beads and the test is positive. In the absence of agglutination, the erythrocytes can pass unhindered through the layer of gel beads and are found at the bottom of the micro-tube after centrifugation. The test is then negative (Figure 3) [14].

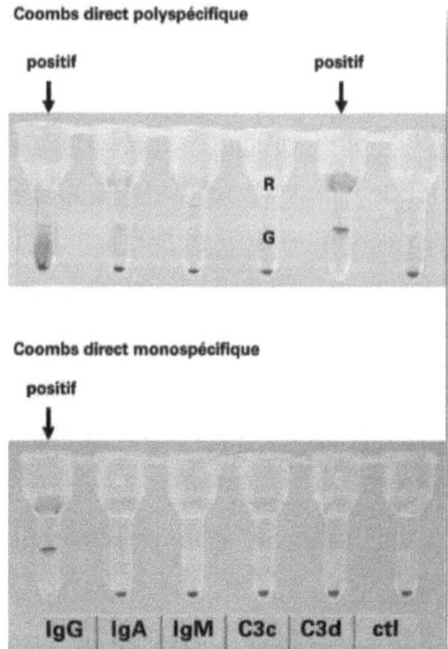

Figure 3: Direct Coombs test in gel [15].

> ➤ The case of biphasic Donath-Landsteiner hemolysin

If TCD is positive with anti-C3d but negative with anti-IgG, a test for cold agglutinins and HBDL should be performed. The Donath Landsteiner (DL) test should be included as a first-line diagnostic test when anemia is accompanied by hemoglobinuria, even if TCD is negative. This test, described by DL almost a hundred years ago, is still the only tool available for diagnosing this form of AHAI. The technique involves incubating patient serum supplemented with fresh AB serum with O RBCs at 4°C for 30 min to allow binding of the AC to the RBCs, followed by a second incubation at 37°C for 1 h to activate complement and produce hemolysis [2]. Thus, the LD test is considered positive when patient serum with or without added complement causes hemolysis only in tubes that have been incubated initially on ice and subsequently at 37°C (figure 4).

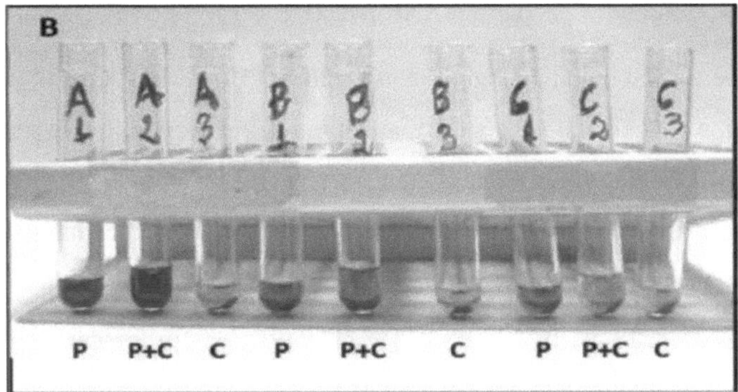

Figure 4: Positive Donath-Landsteiner(DL) test [2].

A: Tubes incubated 30 min at 4°C and 1 h at 37°C; B: Tubes incubated 1 h at 4°C;

C: Tubes incubated 1 h at 37°C; P: patient serum; C: fresh AB serum (source of complement).

2.2.3.2. Serum study

This technique highlights the presence of AAC in serum by bringing it into contact "in vitro" with test RBCs.

The serum study has a triple advantage:

- Demonstrate CA when it is not itself detectable by TCD, for example in cold agglutinin or hot hemolysin syndromes with TCD of the complement type.

- Verify, by comparison with the activity of the eluate and the erythrocyte phenotype of the subject, whether there are several CAs with different specificities and affinities, or an associated allo-CA of transfusion importance which may, in certain circumstances, be solely responsible for TCD positivity.

- Finally, to monitor the evolution of the haematological picture. The reduction and disappearance of serum AAC are the first steps in the remission or cure of AHAI [6].

➢ Search for circulating AACs by TCI :

It can be carried out at a range of temperatures (+4° C, +22° C, +37° C), to determine not only the AAC's thermal optimum, but also its titre. In practice, it is based on the irregular agglutination test (RAI): the patient's serum is brought into contact with a panel of test red blood cells of known phenotype and antiglobulins (anti-IgG and complement). Agglutination indicates the presence of AAC in the serum, whose optimum and/or thermal amplitude can be specified. TCI can also be performed on gel, with sensitivity, specificity, positive predictive value and negative predictive value estimated at 100%, 97.7%, 81.4% and 100% respectively [27]. However, TCI is less sensitive and less specific than TCD (as it is positive in cases of prior alloimmunization), and is not essential for confirming the diagnosis of AHAI [15, 22].

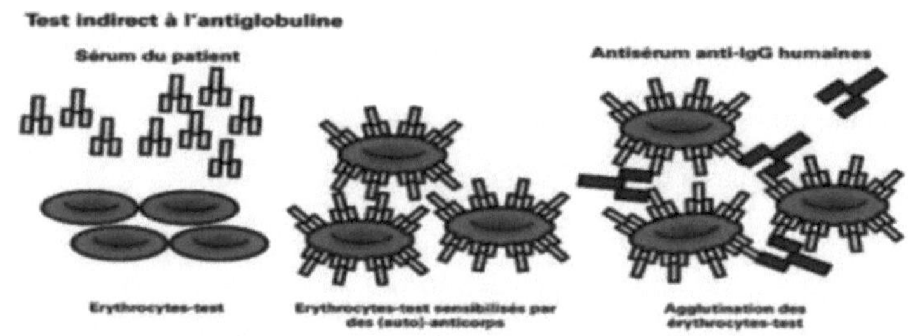

Figure 5: Principle of the indirect Coombs test [15].

➢ Search for circulating AAC in saline :

IgM-type AACs are difficult to detect by TCD, as their size (pentamer) means that they are often washed out during the test. In addition, the thermal amplitude of the CA and the temperature at which the TCI is performed play a decisive role in the detection of IgM-type CAA.

We then exploit the ability of IgM, due to its structure (pentamer) and size, to agglutinate erythrocytes without additional assisting factors (so-called "complete" ACs). Patient serum is incubated at 16 T in the presence of test erythrocytes. Spontaneous agglutination of test erythrocytes indicates the highly probable presence of a "cold" IgM-type CAA.

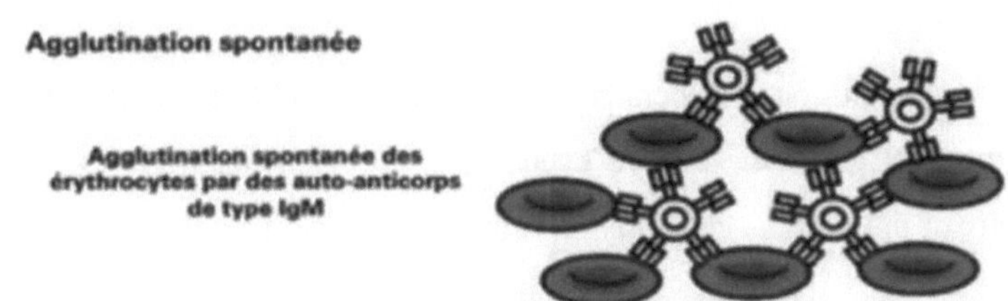

Figure 6: Spontaneous agglutination of erythrocytes by IgM-type AACs [15].

In addition to TCD, the detection of IgM-type hot AACs is based on the study of serum, since the detection of agglutination at temperatures greater than or equal to room temperature, and the absence of this agglutination at lower temperatures, bears witness to this phenomenon. The presence of IgM-type AACs can be confirmed by treatment with DDT (dichlorodiphenyltrichloroethane). DDT inactivates IgM reactivity by reducing the disulfide bonds present in the tertiary structure unique to the IgM pentamer. If IgM AAC is present in the serum, DDT will abolish any spontaneous agglutination of red blood cells [35].

2.2.3.3.   Elution

> Principle

A positive TCD indicates sensitization of red blood cells by CAAs. These CAs can be eluted from RBCs and their specificity determined [15, 36]. Elution can be carried out using a variety of procedures (heating to 56 T, ether, chloroform, xylene, pH lowering, etc.), enabling the collection of CA detached from the RBC surface in a liquid medium, and the study of its reactivity towards the patient's RBCs and an erythrocyte panel, using conventional agglutinin research methods. If the CA agglutinates all the red cells in the panel, it is probably an AAC [36].

A negative elution associated with a positive IgG-type TCD should highlight a possible drug-induced hemolytic anemia, often TCD-positive with a negative elution [2].

In cold AHAI, elution is generally not indicated. AAC can sometimes be eluted from RBCs if these have been stored at +4 T. In this case, the specificity of the AAC is generally reported by the serum study.

2.2.3.4.   Search for associated alloantibodies

DBT is not routinely performed during pre-transfusion testing. However, TCD and additional techniques such as adsoption-elution and titration of CA in the eluate would be beneficial for recently transfused patients [36]. In serum studies, AAC is classically opposed to allo-CA, due to the positivity of the "autologous" control in the former case and the negativity in the latter [14].

In the case of a positive RAI in previously transfused patients, a serum adsorption test on autologous red blood cells is usually necessary to ensure the absence of associated allo-AC in patients who have received transfusions for a period of more than 3 months. A volume of is incubated in the presence of a volume of the patient's serum at 37 T for one hour. The serum is then centrifuged and recovered. After several passages, a conventional IAT is performed using a TCI. However, auto-adsorption is not suitable for recent transfusions or in cases of severe anemia. In such cases, allo-adsorption is preferred, but has the disadvantage of adsorbing allo-ACs directed against high-frequency antigens [22, 36].

2.2.4. Search for pathology associated with AHAI

As part of the etiological diagnosis, we looked for the various pathologies associated with AHAI. The existence of a family history of dysimmunity (first- or second-degree relative), or a personal history, was sought: systemic disease, immune deficiency, autoimmune leukopenia, an abnormal Ig weight assay, a qualitative or quantitative abnormality in cellular immunity, significant elevation of antinuclear factors, etc. The diagnosis of an infection associated with AHAI was based on the study of viral serologies and viral antibody tests. The diagnosis of infection associated with AHAI was based on viral serologies and bacteriological and parasitological examinations for germs responsible for AHAI. In order for a drug to be considered responsible for the onset of HAI, it had to have been previously incriminated in the literature, and have been administered no more than 2 weeks prior to the onset of HAI (appendix).

2.2.5. Evolving criteria

AHAI was considered acute if the hemoglobin (Hb) level was normalized and signs of hemolysis disappeared within 3 months. For chronic AHAI, complete remission was defined by an Hb level above 11 g/dl, and the absence of biological signs of hemolysis for at least 3 months. The mere persistence of a positive DBT was not considered a criterion for non remission. Partial remission was defined as Hb levels of 7 to 11 g/dl and persistence of clinico-biological signs of hemolysis. In all other cases, treatment failure was considered.

2.2.6. Statistical analysis

All data were analyzed using SPSS "Statistical Package for Social Sciences" (version 21). The Chi-squared test or Fisher test was used to compare the frequencies of different patient data. A value of P < 0.05 was considered significant.

3. Results

3.1. Descriptive study

3.1.1. Epidemiological study

3.1.1.1. Annual distribution of AHAI cases

During the ten-year study period (2004-2014), approximately 5993 TCDs were performed at the CRTS for the pediatric department. Of the 25 patients with a positive TCD, we included only 17 for whom we have complete clinico-biological data. 16 cases had isolated AHAI, while only one had Evans syndrome (ES).

The annual incidence of this pathology did not exceed 4 cases per year (Figure 7).

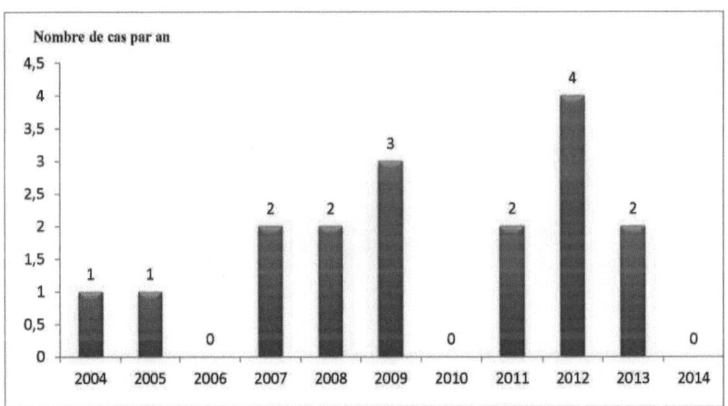

Figure 7: Annual incidence of AHAI (n= 17)

3.1.1.2. Breakdown of our patients by sex

In our series, AHAI affected 7 male patients (41.2%) and 10 female patients (58.8%), with a sex ratio of 0.7 (Figure 8).

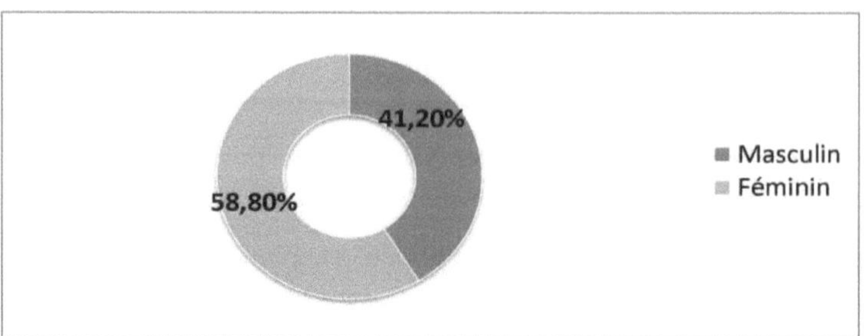

Figure 8: Gender distribution of our patients (n=17)

3.1.1.3.   Age distribution of our patients

Most of our patients (n = 11) were under 4 years of age. Indeed, the average age was 3 years, with extremes ranging from 2 months to 7 years (Figure 9).

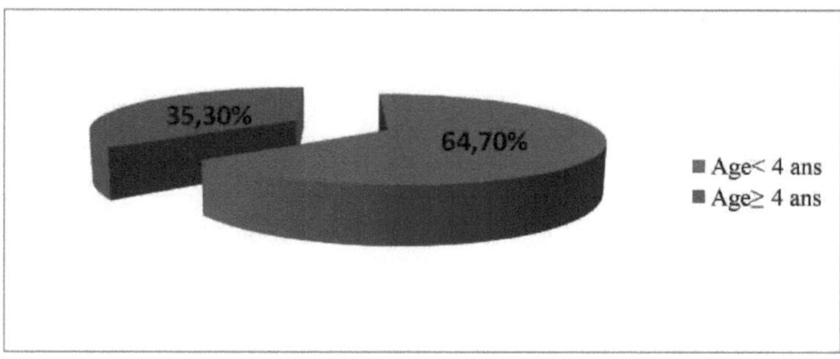

Figure 9: Distribution of patients by age at diagnosis (n=17)

3.1.2. Family survey

3.1.2.1.   Family history

The family survey showed parental consanguinity in 13/17 (76.5%) of our patients (Figure 10).

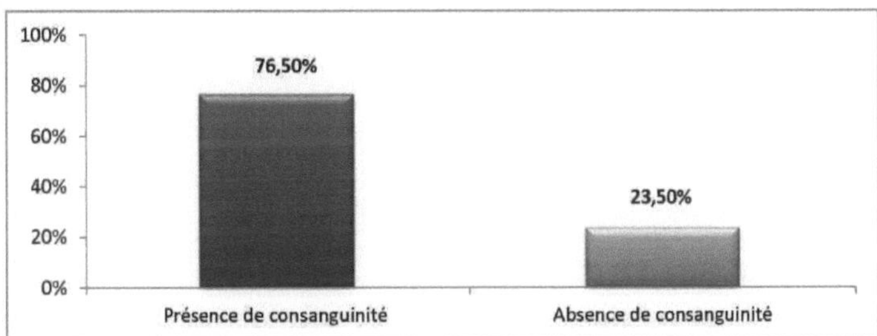

Figure 10: Study of parental consanguinity in our series (n=17)

3.1.2.2.   Personal history

Almost all patients had no personal history of the disease, apart from a single case with both immune deficiency and diabetes (Figure 11).

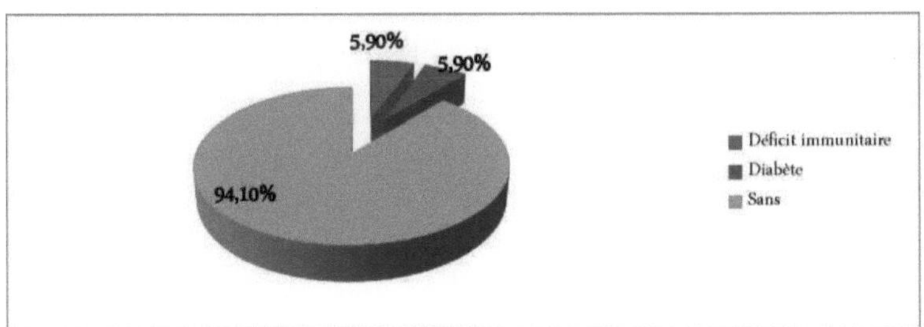

Figure 11: Personal history of our patients (n=17)

3.1.2.3. Transfusion history

In our series, 12/17 patients (70.6%) had received previous transfusions. With the exception of the four beta thalassemics, these transfusions were more than 3 months old (Figure 12).

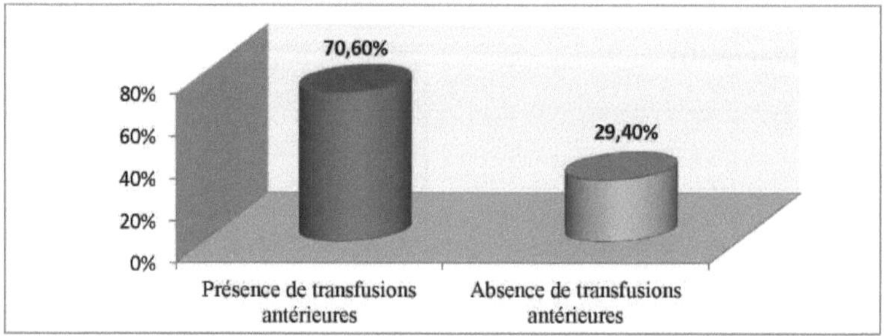

Figure 12: Patients' transfusion history (n=17)

3.1.3. Classification

3.1.3.1. Immunohematological classification

In our patients, we noted a predominance of "hot" type AHAI (88.2%). One patient had a "mixed" AHAI, and in another we suspected either drug-induced AHAI (notion of taking ibuprofen and augmentin), or HBDL (TCD type C3d, cold agglutinin test at +4 T negative, but HBDL test not done) (Figure 13).

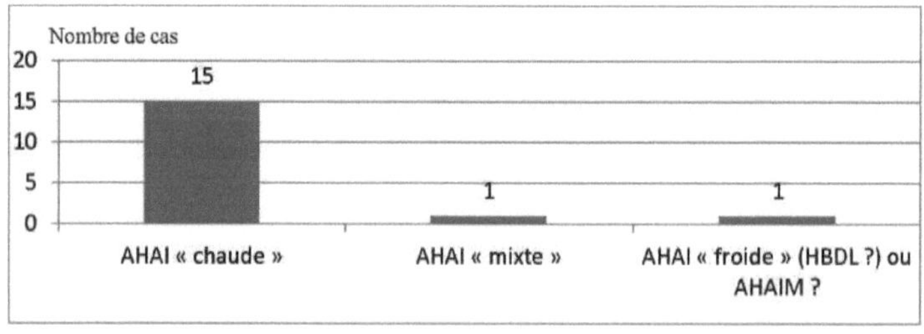

Figure 13: Immunological classification of AHAI cases (n=17)

3.1.3.2. Evolutionary classification

In terms of evolution, our series was equally divided between acute and chronic forms. In only one case was the evolution not specified (Figure 14).

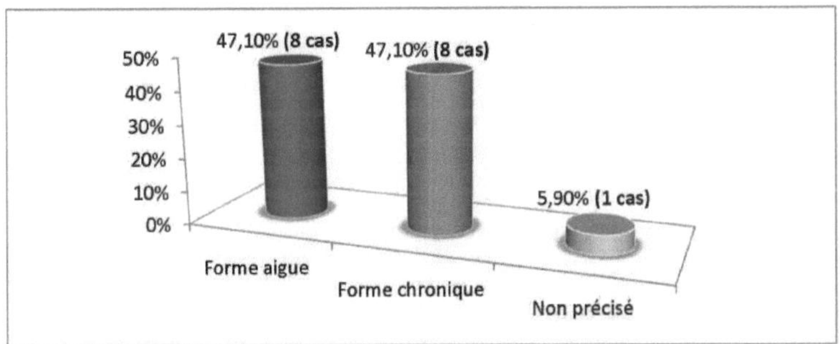

Figure 14: Progressive classification of AHAI cases (n=17)

3.1.3.3. Etiological classification

In our series, a clear predominance of secondary forms was noted in 12/17 (76.47%) of patients, while idiopathic forms presented only (5/17) of cases and included 4 isolated AHAI and 1 SE (Figure 15).

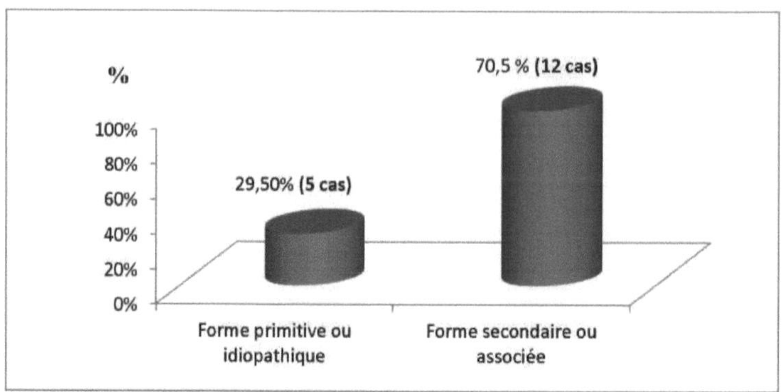

Figure 15: Etiological classification of AHAI cases (n=17)

3.1.4. Clinical diagnosis

3.1.4.1. Circumstances of anaemia discovery

Mucocutaneous pallor was noted in almost all patients on admission (15/17). Jaundice was present in 7/17 cases, and tachycardia in 10/17 cases (Table I).

Table I: Main telltale signs of anemia

	Our series (n =17)	Percentage
Icterus	7	41.17 %
Mucocutaneous heat	15	88.23 %
Exertional dyspnea	2	11.76 %
tachycardia	10	58.82 %

3.1.4.2. Mode of onset of anemia

In 58.8% (10/17) of cases, hemolysis was abrupt, while in the remainder it was progressive (Figure 16).

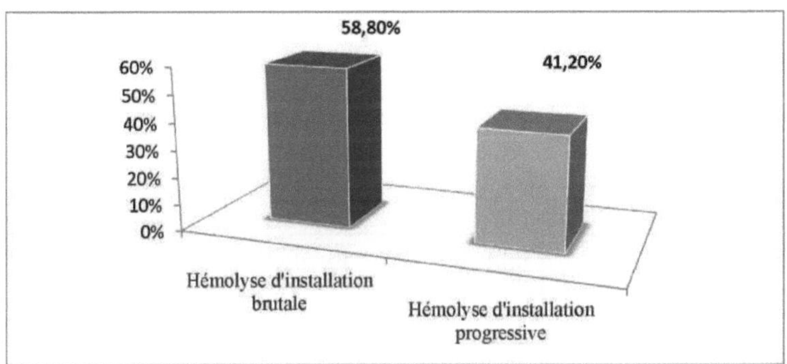

Figure 16: Mode of onset of anemia (n=17)

3.1.4.3. Clinical aspects of the disease

Pallor was noted in all patients. Jaundice was present in 11/17 cases. Hepatomegaly and/or splenomegaly were variable and not always constant. Acrocyanosis, the clinical hallmark of cold AHAI, was absent in all patients (Table II).

Table II: Clinical signs of anemia in our patients

Clinical signs	Our series (n =17)	Percentage
Splenomegaly	10	58.82 %
Hepatomegaly	10	58.82 %
Fever	9	52.94 %
Dark urine	6	35.29
Pallor	17	100 %
jaundice	11	64.7 %
Functional systolic murmur	6	35.29 %

3.1.5. Biological diagnosis

3.1.5.1. Anemia

Anemia was severe, with an Hb level not exceeding 4 g/dl in 4 cases, and moderate in 9 patients (Table III).

Table III: Distribution of Hb levels in our series

Hb level (g/dl)	Number of cases (n =17)	%
<4	4	23,53
4-6	9	52,94
Greater than 6	4	23,53

Anemia was macrocytic in only 3 patients. Bone marrow regeneration was noted in (8/17) cases, whereas (7/17) of our patients had developed aregenerative anemia. In two patients, the reticulocyte count was not determined (Table IV).

Table IV: Characteristics of anemia in our series

Anemia	Number of cases (n =17)	Percentage (%)
Normocytic	10	58,82
Microcytic	4	23,53
Macrocytic	3	17,65
Regenerative	8	47,05
Aregenerative	7	4,17
Not explored	2	11,78

3.1.5.2.   Pancytopenia

Pancytopenia has been described in two patients where AHAI was secondary to visceral leishmaniasis (VL).

3.1.5.3.   Biological signs of hemolysis

Elevated LDH was observed in all cases. Hyperbilirubinemia was noted in 13 patients (76.47%). Haptoglobin levels were measured in only 5 patients, and were always low (Table V).

Table V: Biological signs of hemolysis (n=17)

Biological signs of hemolysis	Average	Min	Max	Usual values
LDH (IU/l)	877	470	3000	200-400
Haptoglobin (g/l)	0,11	0	0,25	0,5-2,5
BNC (pmol/l)	11.32	0	27	< 12

3.1.5.4.   Immunohematological diagnosis

➢ Direct Coombs test

All patients included in our series were TCD positive. It was IgG+C3d in 9/17 (52.94%) and IgG in 7/17 (41.2%) of cases. In only one patient was the TCD complement positive (Figure 17).

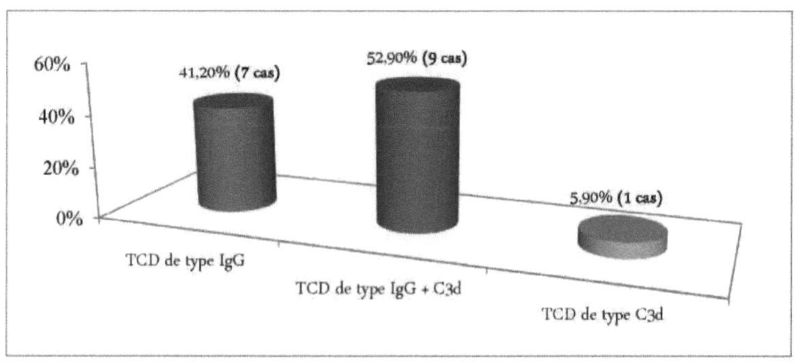

Figure 17: Direct Coombs test results (n=17)

➢ Elution

Direct elution was performed in 8/17 patients. It was positive with an anti-high-frequency antigen specificity, probably from the RH system, in 4/8 (50%) cases, including a single patient in whom the high-frequency AAC disappeared, giving way to an anti-e (1/8) (Figure 18).

> Serum study

Serum studies were carried out in 14/17 of our patients using the indirect
Coombs and enzyme-linked immunosorbent assays, and were positive for
AAC in 8/14 cases (57.14%) (Figure 18). Only one patient (beta thalassemic)
had an allo-AC of specificity "c" associated with AAC. For the case of mixed
AHAI, in addition to the positive indirect Coombs IAA, a saline IAA was
performed with the presence of cold agglutinins (titre of 8; thermal optimum
+4° C).

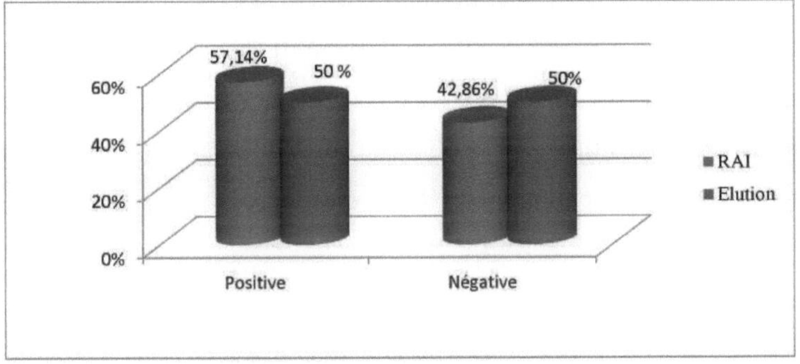

Figure 18: RAI and elution results

3.1.6. Etiological diagnosis

Weighted Ig determination, cellular immunity tests, Hb electrophoresis,
microbiological and parasitological examinations were carried out in search
of disease associated with AHAI. The majority of AHAI cases were post-
infectious (6/17). Beta-thalassemia major was found in 4 patients, immune
deficiency in one and drug-induced AHAI or influenza virus infection
(suspected) in another. Idiopathic forms encompassed 5 cases, including one

SE (Figure 19).

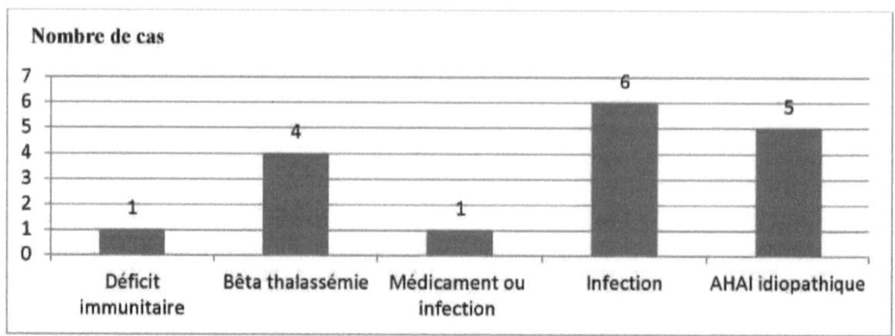

Figure 19: Etiological diagnosis of AHAI in our series (n=17)

In our series, the germs most frequently implicated in AHAI in children were investigated. Most of our patients were tested for viral hepatitis, HIV, cytomegalovirus (CMV), Epstein-Barr virus (EBV) and atypical germs. CMV infection was found in only one patient. It should also be noted that AHAI was secondary to visceral leishmaniasis in 5 patients, and probably associated with an influenza-like illness in only one case. Thus, in our series, infectious etiology accounted for 7/17 cases (Figure 20).

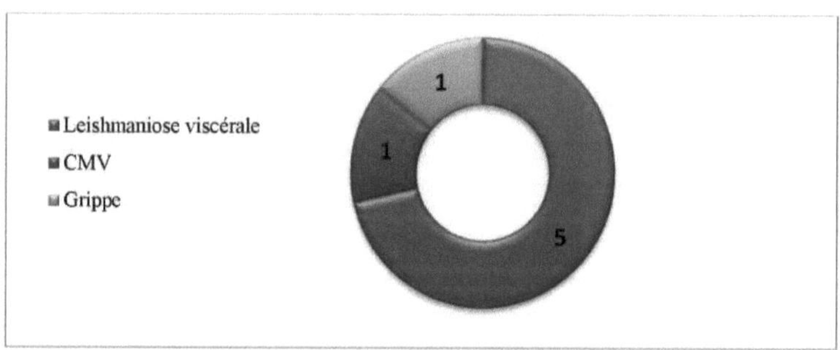

Figure 20: AHAI secondary to infection (n = 7)

3.1.7. Treatment

Almost all patients received blood transfusions (16/17 cases). Corticosteroids were used in 10/17 (58.8%) cases, with adjuvant corticosteroid therapy administered in 7. Only 2 patients received folate supplementation. Splenectomy was performed in only one corticoresistant patient (Figure 21).

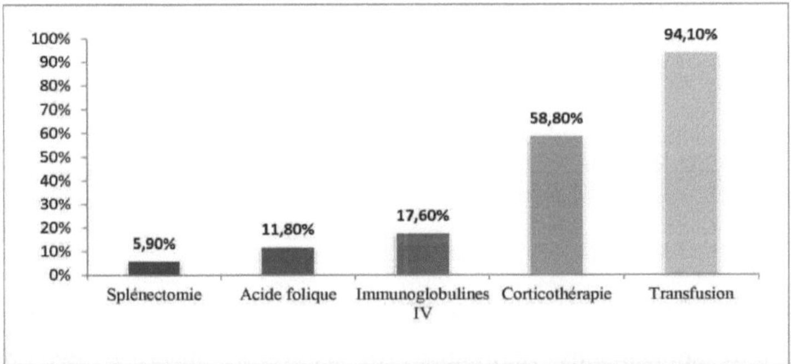

Figure 21: Treatments used in the management of our patients

Transfusion performance was good, moderate and poor in 4/16, 8/16 and 4/16 of cases respectively (Figure 22).

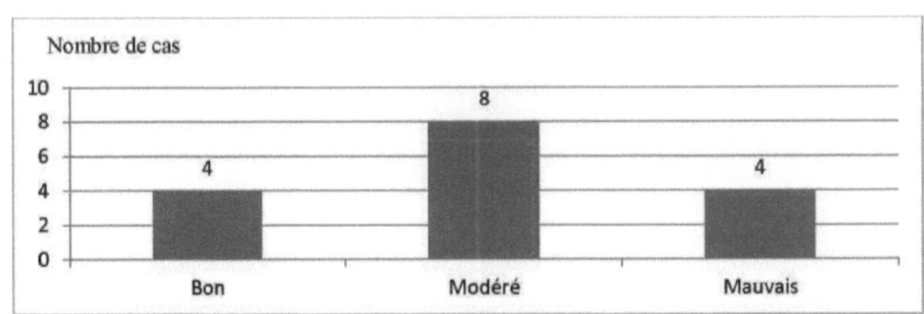

Figure 22: Transfusion efficiency in our patients (n=16)

Corticosteroid therapy was administered in 10/17 patients, and was effective in 4/10 cases; one patient went into remission, then relapsed and was cured on corticosteroid therapy, while two patients became corticoresistant (Figure 23).

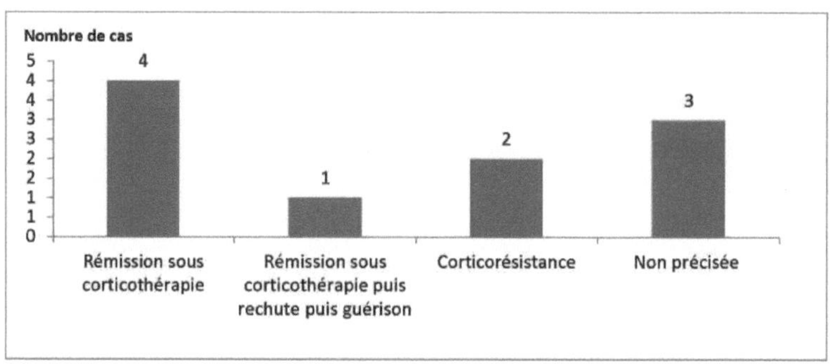

Figure 23: Response to corticosteroid therapy in our patients (n=10)

In all, definitive cure was noted in 9/17 (52.9%) of patients, one of whom went into spontaneous remission. An as yet unspecified evolution encompassed a total of 6/17 (35.3%) cases, who were either lost to follow-up or in the process of being lost to follow-up. Two cases (11.8%) of death were reported (Figure 24).

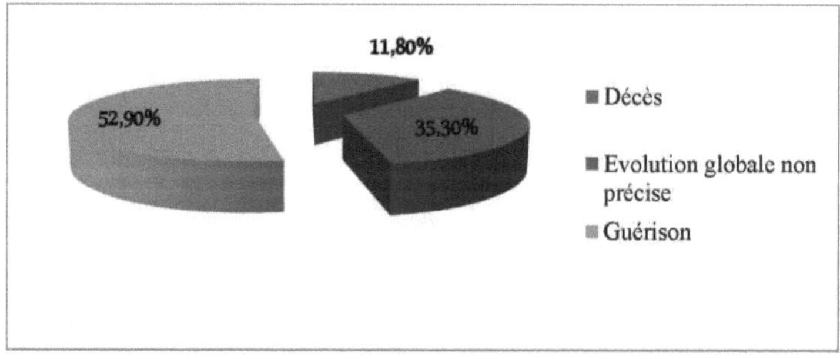

Figure 24: Overall evolution of AHAI in our series (n=17)

3.1.8. Complications

In our series, AHAI-related complications were found in just one patient, who developed dilated cardiomyopathy. Signs of cortisone impregnation were recorded in 3 patients.

3.2.   Analytical study

> Hemolysis in acute transient AHAI (8/17 cases) was abrupt in all cases (100%). In chronic forms (8/17 cases), hemolysis tended to be progressive (87.5%) P = 0.001 (Figure 25).

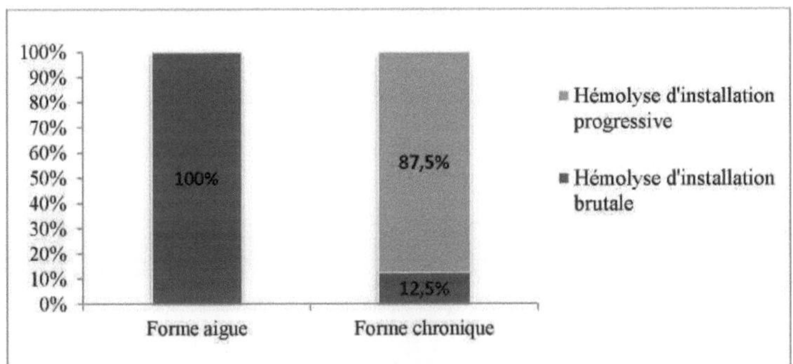

Figure 25: Progressive classification of AHAI according to the mode of onset of hemolysis

> Most patients with acute HAIA (6/8) were under 4 years of age, as were those with chronic HAIA (5/8 cases) (P= 0.84).

> AHAI with IgG + C3d TCD tended to progress to chronicity (62.5%). Patients with C3d TCD tended to have acute AHAI P=0.44 (Figure 26).

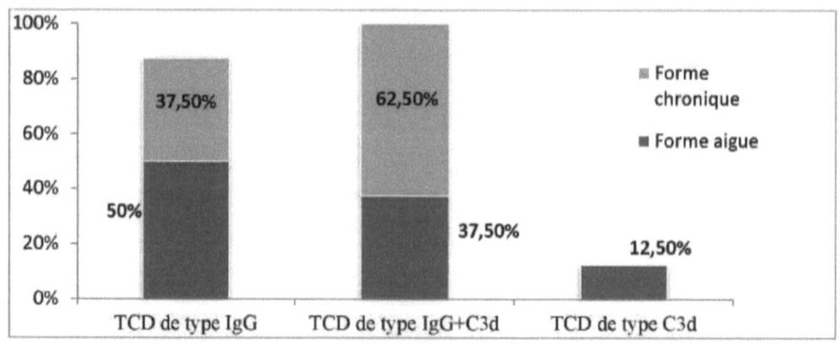

Figure 26: Evolution of AHAI as a function of TCD type

> ➢ In our population, we noted a significant correlation between progressive forms of AHAI and prognosis (P = 0.018). Indeed, 75% (6/8) of acute AHAI evolved towards recovery. In chronic forms, only 3/8 patients (37.5%) were cured (Figure 27).

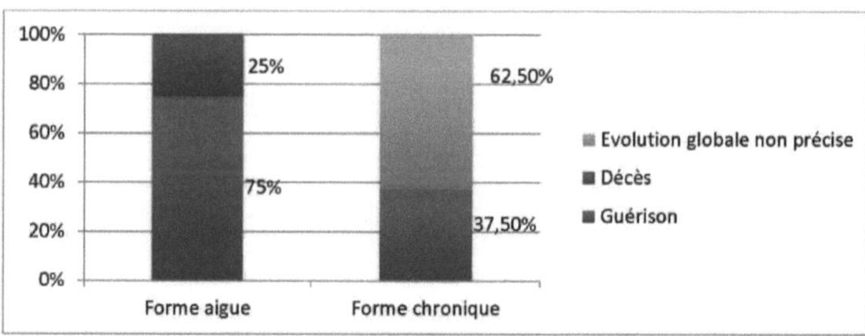

Figure 27: Progressive classification and prognosis of AHAI

> ➢ With the exception of the SE case, which had an unclear overall course, the other idiopathic forms (4 cases) all progressed to cure (100%). Among secondary forms (12 cases), 5/12 (41.6%) of patients were considered cured, while 2 cases of death (AHAI associated with visceral leishmaniasis) were recorded.

P = 0.9 (Figure 28).

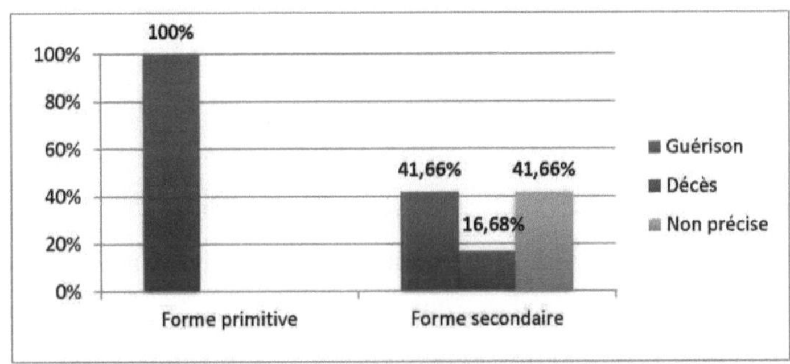

Figure 28: AHAI etiological classification and prognosis

> Patients who did not receive adjuvant corticosteroid therapy were more likely to develop signs of cortisone impregnation. These adverse effects were present in (28.6%) where corticosteroid therapy was used alone versus 10% in whom adjuvant therapy was well conducted. P = 0.53 (Figure 29).

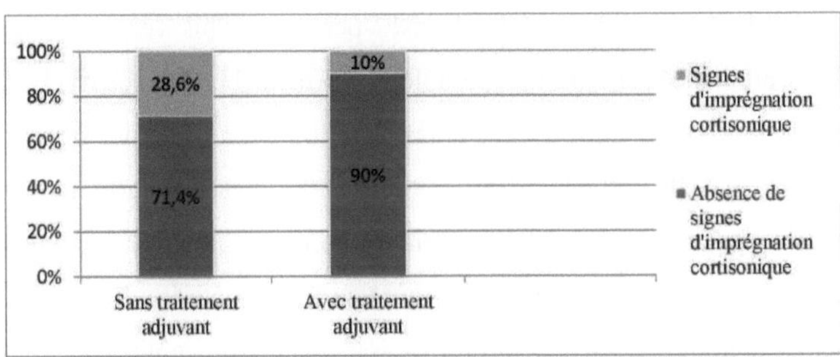

Figure 29: Evaluation of the effect of adjuvant corticosteroid therapy on the appearance of signs of cortisone impregnation.

4. Discussion

The aim of our study was to investigate the epidemiological, clinical-biological, therapeutic and evolutionary profile of AHAI. However, the retrospective nature of the study, the strict inclusion criteria, the rarity of the pathology and the fact that it was limited to a single hospital center and a single clinical department meant that our personal series was numerically modest. Over a period of 10 years (from 2004 to 2014), we were able to collect only 17 cases of AHAI in children, 16 of which were isolated cases, and only one patient with AHAI associated with ITP, known as SE.

4.1. Epidemiology

4.1.1. Frequency

In our series, the number of new cases of AHAI diagnosed in children at EPS Farhat Hached varied from 1 to 4 cases per year. This very low figure confirms published data on this pathology. In fact, this is a relatively rare condition, since epidemiological studies have found an incidence of around 1 to 4 cases per 100,000 inhabitants per year in the Western world, probably lower in the paediatric population, where the incidence is also lower than 0.2 / 100,000 inhabitants. In reality, this figure underestimates its frequency, as it often does not take into account forms associated with another pathology, which is sometimes in the foreground [23, 27, 37]. In 2004, the French Society *of* Hematology *and Immunology (SHIP)* launched a national observatory of children with AHAI, which ran until December 2007. During this period, the number of new cases per year varied from 15 to 35, confirming the rarity of this pathology [30].

4.1.2. Age

In our patients, the mean age at diagnosis was 3 years, with a clear predominance of AHAI before the age of 4 (11/17 cases). This is in line with the literature, which reports that AHAI can occur at any age, although it is rarer in children than in adults. They mainly affect children under the age of 4 and adults over the age of 40. Indeed, the largest paediatric series estimate that over 60% are under 4 years of age, with a median age of diagnosis of 3.7 years [12, 17, 28]. A retrospective study carried out at the immuno-hematological unit of the "La Sapienza" University of Rome blood bank between 1986 and 2003 showed that the peak incidence of AHAI was in the first 4 years of life [38]. Similarly, in the prospective study by the French Society of Hematology and Immunology, AHAI was more frequent before the age of 4, with 21% (57/265) under the age of 1 [30]. This frequent occurrence of AHAI before the age of 4 and after the age of 40 could be due, respectively, to the predominance of transient acute forms in children and the increased frequency of chronic forms and lymphoproliferative malignancies in the elderly [17, 39].

4.1.3. Gender

Our study showed a predominance of females (58.8%) with a sex ratio of 0.7. The study in children by Tantawy et al. also showed that among 32 children with AHAI, 25 (78%) were girls [40]. However, according to other paediatric series, such as that of Habibi et al [6], this predominance is reversed and becomes more male. Similarly, Vaglio et al [38] found in their study a sex ratio close to unity (51 boys and 49 girls). This variability in gender distribution remains poorly explained. In addition, in adulthood, AHAI is characterized by a discrete female predominance. The male/female ratio is 0.5 to 0.6 [16, 30].

4.1.4. Genetic factors and family history

In our series, we found familial consanguinity in 13/17 (76.5%) patients, although no familial cases of AHAI were detected. The existence of a hereditary component in the development of AHAI is a controversial subject. Several early publications reported multiple familial cases of AHAI, underlining the existence of a certain genetic predisposition to the development of autoimmune disorders (Table VI):

Table VI: Published family cases of AHAI [6].

Authors	Affected family members
Kissmeyer-Nielsen et al	Mother and daughter
Dobbs	Two brothers and a sister
Shapiro	Five brothers and sisters
Zuelzer et al	Two monozygotic twins.
Jensen et al.	Five brothers and sisters
Habibi et al.	Monozygotic twins Mother and son

On the other hand, until 2010, some authors maintained that these publications had no genetic basis, arguing that AHAI has no known predisposition, no age preselection, and no familial hereditary component [18]. In 2011, Aladjidi et al. did identify a genetic predisposition and immune disorders underlying AHAI. Their French national cohort is known as the largest series of childhood AHAIs, given the scope of the study they conducted (265 children) and the systematic collection of family data on patients [30].

In our series, we found no cases of AHAI with a family history of autoimmune disorders. According to the previously cited French cohort, familial immunological pathologies were identified in 15^0 % (41/265) of cases [30].

4.2. Clinical diagnosis

4.2.1. How anemia develops

In our series, hemolysis was abrupt in onset in 10/17 cases (58.8%), resulting in 2 deaths. In the remaining patients, the onset of symptoms was progressive. Moreover, we noted a significant correlation between the progressive forms of AHAI and the mode of onset of anemia (P= 0.001). Indeed, in all acute forms of AHAI (8/8), hemolysis was abrupt. In chronic forms, on the other hand, hemolysis was mainly progressive (7/8 cases). Our results are supported by the publications of Habibi et al (Table VII).

Table VII: Evolution of AHAI according to the mode of onset of haemolysis in the series by Habibi et al [41].

	Habibi et al. series	
	Acute AHAI (N=34)	Chronic AHAI (N= 46)
Sudden onset of hemolysis	21	15
Progressive hemolysis	13	31

4.2.2. Clinical aspects

The symptomatology of AHAI depends on the rapidity and intensity of hemolysis [6]. In our study, the main clinical manifestations of the disease noted in our patients are very similar to those described in the literature (Table VIII).

Table VIII: Clinical signs of AHAI in our patients compared with other paediatric series

Clinical signs of AHAI	Egyptian retrospective study (n =32) [40]	Habibi.B et al series (n= 80) [41]	Our study (n =17)
Splenomegaly	17	44	10
Hepatomegaly	17	24	10
Fever	11	-	9
Icterus	26	70	11
Pallor	32	65	17
Acrocyanosis	-	-	0
Hemoglobinuria	-	2	-

In the literature, in young children, the disease is often described as preceded by a non-specific fever. In all cases, the child shows conjunctival pallor and jaundice on examination. Splenomegaly is typical of "hot" AHAI, while hemoglobinuria or acrocyanosis is suggestive of "cold" AHAI [2]. Garrett F. Bass et al. have reported that these clinical signs can sometimes be overshadowed by underlying diseases In the case of HPF, after a few minutes to a few hours of exposure to cold, the patient usually develops abdominal cramps, headache, often followed by chills and fever. The first urine after the onset of symptoms usually contains Hb [10].

In certain circumstances, AHAI can be asymptomatic. Indeed, McGann et al. reported the case of a one-year-old girl who developed IgA-type CDT

AHAI. The patient was clinically asymptomatic, with normal vital signs, no pallor, jaundice or hepatosplenomegaly. Anemia was discovered incidentally during a routine laboratory examination showing an Hb level of 9 g/dl [42].

4.3. Biological diagnosis

4.3.1. Blood count

In our series, anemia was severe (Hb <4 g/dl) in 4/17 patients, while more than half (9/17) had moderate anemia (Hb 4-6 g/dl). Anemia was normocytic, macrocytic and microcytic in 10/17, 3/17 and 4/17 cases respectively. The literature reports that Hb values are highly variable, ranging from low to high. Biologically, the diagnosis of AHAI is evoked by anaemia that is classically normochromic, macrocytic and regenerative. However, it should be noted that these biological signs may be absent or abolished by underlying pathologies associated with AHAI [22, 23, 34] [22]. Spinal cord regeneration, a situation normally expected in this pathology, was found in only 8/17 (47.05%) of our patients. Similarly, Aladjid et al. found that 45/223 children had a reticulocyte count below 100,000 at diagnosis [12].

Patients with aregenerative AHAI (7 cases) in our series did not receive folate supplementation, and Hb levels did not exceed 6 g/dl. In 6/7 of these cases, AHAI was secondary to another pathology: visceral leishmaniasis (1 case), immune deficiency (1 case), beta-thalassemia major (4 cases). Indeed, data from the literature suggest that most cases of reticulocytopenia are observed in patients whose bone marrow function is depressed by underlying pathologies, infections, toxic chemicals or nutritional deficiency. Such patients may rapidly develop severe anemia, and early transfusion may be indicated [17].

Although the erythrocyte response in "hot" AHAI is variable, the reticulocyte count is generally high and when it exceeds 20%, AHAI will be very likely, but a normal or even lowered reticulocyte count can nevertheless be observed in 10 to 20% of AHAI cases and this in 3 situations:

- In the very early stages of AHAI, hyperreticulocytosis may be delayed by a few days.

- When AACs are directed against antigens common to mature erythrocytes and reticulocytes and/or erythroblasts.

- In cases of associated folate deficiency [4, 22, 34].

4.3.2. Biological haemolysis syndrome

The hemolytic nature of the anemia in our patient was easily identified by the moderate elevation of LDH (100% of cases) and/or unconjugated bilirubin (UB) (76.4% of cases) and especially by the drop in haptoglobin in all cases where it was tested.

Despite the fact that all our patients had fairly high LDH levels, elevated LDH levels are inconsistent with the diagnosis of AHAI (80%) [29].

When present, free hyperbilirubinemia is highly suggestive of HA [17].

In our study, only five patients had a haptoglobin assay, which was found to be low. In fact, the Hb released into the plasma following hemolysis binds to haptoglobin, its transport protein. The constant decrease in haptoglobin is confirmed as the most sensitive marker of hemolysis (95% sensitivity in the absence of associated inflammatory syndrome) [17, 22, 27, 29].

4.3.3. Immunohematological diagnosis of AHAI

4.3.3.1. Direct Coombs test

All patients included in our series had a positive TCD.

Some authors suggest that TCD, the cornerstone of diagnosis, is positive in 95% of cases of AHAI. It is both necessary and sufficient to confirm the autoimmune nature of HA [27]. However, according to the literature, TCD positivity is a necessary but not sufficient condition for the diagnosis of AHAI [27].

In fact, a positive DBT is found in 0.5 to 8% of hospitalized patients, even when there is no HA, and in 1.4% of healthy subjects. Thus, if a test is positive, it must be interpreted according to the clinical context [33, 36].

In our series, TCD revealed a predominance of AHAI with IgG + C3d/ IgG type TCD found in 16/17 cases. Only one case of C3d type was reported. This predominance of IgG+C3d/IgG forms was also reported by Aladjidi et al (Table X).

Table IX: Type of TCD (our series / series by Aladjidi et al.) [30]

TCD type	Nathalie Aladjidi et al	Our series
Ig G	42 %	41.2 %
IgG +C3d	32 %	52.9 %
C3d	24 %	5.9 %
Ig A	1 %	-

According to early publications, in the pediatric population, the vast majority of post-infectious AHAIs were associated with complement-type CDT with or without elevated cold agglutinins, whereas chronic forms were accompanied by IgG or mixed-type CDT[41] . This concept was subsequently challenged by Aladjidi and colleagues, who showed that in 74% of cases studied, the CDT was IgG/IgG+C3d (Table X) [30]. Based on the type of TCD and the thermal optimum, we were able to distinguish 2 classes of AHAI, namely "hot" AHAI (15/17) and "mixed" AHAI (1/17). However, in the case where the TCD was C3d with absence of cold agglutinins at +4 T negative, we were unable to distinguish between cold AHAI (HBDL: biological test not performed) and AHAIM (notion of taking buprofen and augmentin with spontaneously favorable evolution on discontinuation of treatment). This predominance of the hot form in children in our series has also been found in other studies, as shown in Table XI.

Table X: AHAI classification (our series / Vaglio series / Sokol series).

	Series Vaglio et al n= 100 [38]	Sokol et al series n= 42 [43]	Our series n= 17
Hot" AHAI	64	16	15
Cold AHAI — AHAI with cold agglutinins	26	5	0
Cold AHAI — HBDL	6	17	1 suspected
Mixed" AHAI	4	4	1

4.3.3.2. Elution

In our series, 8/17 patients underwent elution. However, given the pitfalls and technical parameters involved, positivity was only found in half of the cases, all of whom had presented AACs with high-frequency anti-antigen specificity, probably from the RH system. In one patient, at some point during follow-up, we noted a transient shift from public anti-antigen specificity to anti-e specificity. This is not surprising, since frequent changes in the nature and specificity of AACs can occur during the course of the disease [6]. In addition, IgG AACs generally have anti-RH specificity, the least rare specificity remaining the "e" specificity, but most often the AAC is directed against the public antigen carried by all red blood cells of normal RH phenotype [44]. In addition to the RH system, other antigens of certain blood group systems can be the target of AAC (anti-LW^a , anti-LW^{ab} , anti-S, anti-U, anti-En^a , anti-Wr^b , antiGerbich, anti-M, anti-N, anti-Pr) [14].

Vaglio and colleagues reported that direct elution was negative in cases of negative TCD or positive complement alone. They also demonstrated that when elution was positive, eluted AACs had clear specificity in only 5 cases of warm AHAI, namely: anti-e (3/5), anti-D (1/5), anti-Ce (1/5) [38]. Although anti-D specificity has already been cited by Vaglio, Bercovitz et al. recently claimed exclusive responsibility for the discovery of a case of primary IgG AAC "hot" AHAI with anti-D specificity in a one-year-old patient [32]. In Tunisia, Oucheri et al. identified an autoAC with anti-D specificity in an adult with a D type 4.0 phenotype, followed for a myelodysplastic syndrome and regularly treated with transfusions [45].

Anti-Jk specificity[a] has rarely been described. It was only in 2013 that Giovannetti et al. reported the case of a 5-year-old girl who developed "hot" AHAI associated with Parvovirus B19 infection, the identified AAC being of anti Jk specificity[a] [31].

4.3.3.3. Serum study

Serum may contain antibodies not fully adsorbed to RBCs. In our patients, 14 cases were tested for AAC. The test was positive for AAC, with pan-agglutination in 8/14 patients. Only one patient, known to be beta thalassemic, had developed an allo-AC of anti-c specificity associated with AAC. The presence of associated allo-AC in AHAI is not an uncommon occurrence. Indeed, the pediatric study by Vaglio et al. reported that allo-ACs were also present in the serum of 5/100 regularly transfused patients with secondary AHAI. The specificity of these allo-ACs was respectively: anti-e, anti-E, antiK, anti-C + anti-Kpa, Anti-E + anti-JKb + anti-S + anti-K [38].

4.4. Etiological diagnosis

4.4.1. Infections

Infections are classically associated with transient acute forms of AHAI. Some of these have been clearly identified, but many AHAIs are associated with unlabelled infectious conditions [14].

4.4.1.1. Viral infections

Although viral etiology is a predominant cause of AHAI in en fant, we found only one case of CMV infection. AHAI associated with CMV infection has also been reported in the literature. Saeko Kaneko et al. described the case of a 1-year-old Japanese boy with TCD-negative AHAI associated with CMV infection [46]. In addition, Tantawy et al. showed that among 13 CMV serologies performed in their studies, 7 were positive [40]. In our series, another viral etiology (influenza) was retained without serological proof, given the existence of an infectious context preceding the hemolytic crisis. Influenza infection has rarely been implicated in the occurrence of AHAI [47]. Indeed, 2 cases have been reported respectively by Chen et al [48] and Schoindre et al [49].

In the literature, the viral etiologies most frequently associated with AHAI are infectious mononucleosis (IM) and viral hepatitis [14, 50]. Hemolytic anemia is present in 1-3% of cases of IM. It most often involves IgM-type cold agglutinins with anti-i specificities [50]. AHAI has also been frequently reported in association with hepatitis A, B and C [20, 51], and it was not until 2009 that Pandey and colleagues [52] reported the case of a 9-year-old girl who developed AHAI with a spontaneously favorable course following infection with hepatitis E virus.

In our series, HIV (human immunodeficiency virus) serology was negative in 14/17 cases. According to the literature, AHAI rarely complicates HIV infection, although TCD positivity in HIV-infected patients is estimated at 20-40%, and this test is rarely accompanied by hemolysis [53].

Our patients were not tested for varicella. In fact, AHAI is a rare complication of chickenpox. This association has been reported in an 11-year-old girl, with a favorable outcome under corticosteroid treatment [37].

Moreover, in the recent French cohort, multiple viral etiologies were described. Indeed, in 22% (49/219) of microbiologically investigated cases, the initial diagnosis of AHAI was concomitant with a well-defined infection: EBV (n = 11), parvovirus (N = 5), rotavirus (n = 4), human herpes virus 6 (n = 3), adenovirus (N = 1), human herpes virus 1 (n = 1), and enterovirus (n = 1) [30].

4.4.1.2.   Bacterial infections

In our series, we found no cases of AHAI secondary to bacterial infection. However, in the literature, this etiology plays a predominant role in AHAI in children, essentially mycoplasma pneumonia associated with cold agglutinins, and syphilis [14, 40, 54].

4.4.1.3.   Parasites

In our patients, the search for an infectious parasitic etiology revealed a predominance of AHAI associated with visceral leishmaniasis, affecting five of the six post-infectious cases. Although anemia is a common finding, TCD-positive AHAI has rarely been reported with VL [55, 56]. Activation of the complement pathway by the formation of circulating antigen-AC complexes is thought to be the most likely mechanism [57].

The AHAI-LV association was first described in 1930 [58]. Since then, further publications have been reported in the paediatric population, mainly involving patients in leishmaniasis-endemic regions such as India, Bangladesh, Nepal and Sudan [55, 56, 58].

Teulade et al. also reported the case of a 3-year-old girl who contracted VL with ACC production, and whose evolution was favorable under treatment with liposomal amphotericin [59].

Few Tunisian studies are available on this subject, but the team of Braham et al. at the Fattouma Bourguiba Hospital in Monastir reported a case of VL associated with AHAI in an 18-year-old adolescent with IgG-positive TCD [57].

Because of the rich and unspecific nature of its clinical manifestations, VL can mimic a systemic disease, and it is therefore possible that patients with VL, wrongly diagnosed as having an autoimmune disease, could be treated with immunosuppressive drugs with potentially fatal consequences. Diagnosis of VL is easy, as long as it is considered, which avoids a large number of unnecessary or aggressive investigations [58, 59].

None of our patients had presented with AHAI secondary to malaria, although AHAI is a complication frequently encountered in malaria, particularly with *Plasmodium falciparum* and *Plasmodium vivax*. [60, 61]. Until 2013, no case of AHAI associated with *Plasmodium. ovale* infection had been reported. Since then, this association has been described in a 3-year-old child from sub-Saharan Africa [62].

4.4.2. AHAI associated with other autoimmune manifestations

Association with other autoimmune manifestations has mainly been reported in the setting of "hot" AHAI [14]. In our series, we found no cases secondary to systemic lupus erythematosus (SLE); however, only one patient had idiopathic SE. The latter corresponds to the association of AHAI and autoimmune thrombocytopenic purpura (ITP) occurring simultaneously or in succession. Our results are confirmed by data in the literature, since the most frequently reported conditions, particularly in children, are SLE and SE [15, 63].

In the Egyptian retrospective study [40] and the French cohort [30], SE was found in 50% and 37% of children respectively. In contrast, the studies by

H. Eddou et al [33] and Chi Young et al [64] reported that SE is a relatively rare condition found in less than 1% of patients with ITP and less than 5% of patients with AHAI. Certain difficulties may arise in daily practice, leading to overdiagnosis of this entity. H. Eddou et al. have pointed out that the presence of cytopenias in an immunological context is not sufficient to make the diagnosis of ES. Myelodysplastic syndromes, for example, when associated with cytopenias of peripheral origin, may pose a differential diagnosis problem with ES [33].

On the other hand, Nathalie Aladjidi et al. reported in their series 3 cases of AHAI associated with SLE. The diagnosis of SLE was made after the discovery of AHAI [30].

4.4.3. Immune deficiency

In our series, humoral immunity was investigated in 9 patients and cellular immunity in 4. We found only one case of AHAI secondary to immune deficiency, the patient being a carrier of Kostman syndrome (congenital neutropenia).

According to the literature, constitutional (and acquired) immune deficiencies predispose to AHAI [12]. Of the various types of immune deficiency, three are more likely to give rise to autoimmune manifestations: common variable immunodeficiency (CVID), SLPA and isolated IgA deficiency. Indeed, in addition to recurrent infections, patients with CVID are at increased risk of developing autoimmune pathologies, including AHAI (2.8% to 6.4% of cases) [63, 65, 66].

4.4.4. Hereditary haemoglobin abnormalities

In our series, AHAI was secondary to an inherited Hb abnormality in 4 patients (23.5%), all with beta thalassemia major.

This association is well established in the literature. Vaglio et al. described it in 5/100 patients, 4 of whom had beta-thalassemia major, the fifth had associated sickle cell disease [38].

Anti-erythrocyte autoimmunization is a frequently reported immune dysfunction in polytransfused patients [66]. A prospective study in Tunisia involving 130 regularly transfused beta-thalassemic patients showed that 40% of patients developed a positive CDT, while AHAI was detected in only 21% of patients [67].

AACs may be of the cold or warm type. They are most often associated with the existence of anti-erythrocytic allo-AC [66]. Thus, it has been reported that the frequency of this association varies from 25 to 30% in thalassemias and from 8 to 45% in major sickle cell syndromes [66]. In our study, only one beta thalassemic patient had developed allo-AC (anti-c) associated with AAC.

On the other hand, other authors suggest that anti-erythrocyte autoimmunization and the development of AHAI could be a complication of allogeneic RBC transfusion [38].

4.4.5. Solid tumors

None of our patients had a solid tumour. However, in all the different published series of childhood AHAI, various solid tumors have been reported. Cure of the AHAI after removal of the tumour suggests the existence of a link between the two, hence the importance of looking for an associated tumour. In the literature, the most frequently reported are teratomas of the ovary, thymomas and gastric tumours [14, 68, 69, 70].

4.4.6. Hematological malignancies

In our series, we found no cases of AHAI secondary to haematological malignancy. This is probably due to the fact that such pathologies are recruited to the clinical hematology department.

Moreover, according to the literature, unlike in adults, malignant disease is rarely revealed or accompanied by AHAI in children [12, 14].

According to a retrospective study covering the last 25 years, carried out in 2011 among member centers of the French Society of Child and Adolescent Cancers (SFCE), among 11 children with Hodgkin's disease, one had with associated AHAI and the other SE [11].

Furthermore, in adults, the clinical course of chronic lymphocytic leukemia (CLL) can be complicated at any time by autoimmune phenomena [71], including AHAI, with a frequency ranging from 4.5% to 11% [71,72]. Indeed, Moreno et al. reported that among 960 CLL patients, 6% were complicated by AHAI and 0.1% by SE [74]. Similarly, Zent and Kay found a 2.3% incidence of CLL complicated by AHA [75].

4.4.7. Drug-induced AHAI (AHAIM)

In our series, AHAI secondary to medication was suspected in only one case. The patient had received ibuprofen and augmentin for 15 days to treat recurrent episodes of influenza. The dark appearance of the urine and jaundice disappeared on discontinuation of treatment. The involvement of ibuprofen, penicillin and beta-lactam inhibitors in the development of AHAI has been reported in the literature [4]. Indeed, a recent study dating from 2013, focused on the incrimination of ibuprofen in a patient suffering from AHAI. Progressive hematological recovery was obtained within 3 days of stopping this treatment [76].

AHAIM has an incidence of one case per million inhabitants and can have a fatal course. Bollotte et al. have shown that this form of AHAI can occur in both children and adults, regardless of sex [21]. Vaglio.S et al. have reported that, in children, drugs are less frequently associated with AHAI, probably because most drugs that can induce AHAI, such as alpha-methyldopa in the past, are not prescribed in children. When they do occur, AHAIMs in children are generally due to IgG-type AACs and are most often associated with antibiotics such as penicillin [38].

The first case of AHAIM was reported in 1950. The number of drugs causing AHAI has evolved considerably, from 30 in 1980 to 130 in 2011 [4, 71]. Among this impressive number of drugs that can cause AHAI are those that can be administered in children: penicillin, cefixime, beta-lactamase inhibitors, furosemide, ibuprofen, mefenamic acid, insulin, isoniazid, methotrexate, teicoplanin, rifampicin, ticarcillin, vancomycin, etc. [21, 77-79].

4.4.8. New associations

MYH9 syndrome is an autosomal dominant disorder caused by a mutation in the MYH9 gene on chromosome 22, coding for the NMMHC-IIA5 *(non muscle myosin heavy chain IIA)* protein. The diagnosis may be suspected on examination of the blood smear, which reveals macroplatelets associated with leukocyte inclusions known as "pseudo Dhole bodies". The first case of association of AHAI with MYH9 syndrome was reported in 2012 in a 28-year-old man. It suggests an incidental association, but serves as a reminder of the importance of blood smear analysis in the setting of hemolysis with thrombocytopenia [80].

4.5. Treatment of AHAI

The management of AHAI depends first and foremost on its tolerance, which in turn depends on the rapidity of onset and severity of the hemoglobin fall, as well as on the underlying condition [13].

4.5.1. Hot" AHAI treatment

4.5.1.1.   Corticosteroid therapy

Corticosteroid therapy is generally prescribed at a dose of 1 to 2 mg/kg/d of prednisone equivalent for 3 to 4 weeks. In the event of an initial response, the dose is then reduced in a slowly progressive manner for a total duration varying according to the authors from 4 to 12 months after remission has been achieved. It seems that a period of 3 to 4 weeks is necessary and sufficient to judge the efficacy of corticosteroid therapy [13, 14, 16].

In our series, corticosteroid therapy was administered as first-line treatment in 10 patients (58.8%), 4 of whom (40%) proved to be corticosteroid-sensitive, achieving remission on this treatment, while two others developed corticoresistance. Our results are similar to those of the Egyptian retrospective study, in which 15/32 (46.9%) of patients had a complete response to corticosteroids after 1 month. However, some authors have found that the response rate to corticosteroids is in the order of 70-80% in 1-3 weeks [2, 12].

In the prospective French study, Aladjid et al. reported that 41% (86/209) of patients on corticosteroid therapy required second-line treatment, due to cortico-dependence or cortico-resistance [12]. These findings were also supported by the publication of Michel M, who asserted that some 60-70% of initially responsive patients relapse if treatment is prematurely discontinued, thus becoming cortico-dependent [22].

Despite the diversity of figures expressing the response rate to corticosteroid therapy, according to the data in the literature, this therapeutic modality remains the first-line treatment essentially for "warm" IgG AHAI, including those secondary to lymphoid hematological malignancies, for which specific treatment is unnecessary [2, 12].

4.5.1.2.   Splenectomy

In our series, splenectomy was performed as a second-line treatment in a single corticoresistant patient, but remained ineffective on the evolution of AHAI. This could be explained by the location of RBC sequestration, probably in the liver, despite the fact that the patient had a warm AHAI with IgG-type AAC.

According to the literature, splenectomy is effective as a second- or third-line treatment in 60% of cases, but only if the AAC is warm and red cell destruction occurs preferentially in the spleen [2, 13, 14]. Habibi.B et al. considered splenectomy as a second-line treatment for corticoresistance or corticodependence in 16/46 patients with chronic AHAI. After an average follow-up of 3 years, complete disappearance of hemolysis was observed in 8/16 patients (50%) [41].

The major risk of splenectomy in children, especially infants, is infection by encapsulated microorganisms. Prior to this procedure, the child must receive vaccinations against pneumococcus, meningococcus and *Haemophilus Influenzae*. In addition, one or two prophylactic doses of oral penicillin should be administered daily for a period of at least 5 years [2].

4.5.1.3.   Rituximab (Mabthera®)

Probably because of its very high cost, none of our corticoresistant patients benefited from rituximab-based treatment, which is a genetically engineered chimeric monoclonal anti-CD20 AC recognizing the CD20 antigen present on B lymphocytes. It has been used successfully in refractory AHAI and in patients unsuitable for splenectomy [12, 63, 81]. Indeed, Giulino et al [81] have reported that, in children and in the face of non-response to conventional therapies, Rituximab has been used successfully, giving complete responses in around 92% of cases. In adults, the response rate did not exceed 54%. Rituximab therefore appears to be more effective in treating this condition in children than in adults. However, Stasi et al [82] have reported that in adults and children treated with this agent, the clinical response is around 85%. The success rate does not seem to depend on the number of previous treatments (including splenectomy), the type of CA or the form of AHAI [83].

Since 2008, several studies have highlighted the earlier use of anti-CD20 to treat this pathology as quickly as possible (Tables XIII and XIV).

Table XI: Use of rituximab in warm agglutinin AHAI [23].

Years	Number of cases	Full answer	Partial response	Second line	Third line
2002	2	0/2	0/2		+
2003	5	2/5			+
2007	1		1/1	+	
2007	11	8/11	3/11		+
2009	27	8/27	17/27		+
2009	53	44/53		+	
2010	36	28/36	6/36	+	+

Table XII: Use of rituximab or new drugs in cold agglutinin AHAI (cold agglutinin disease) [23].

Years	Medicines	Number of cases	Full answer	Partial response	Long-term trend
2002	Rituximab	2	2/2		Good
2009	Eculizumab(anti-C5)	1	1/1		
2010	Rituximab	29	6/29	16/29	Good

Based on these studies, D. Rigal and F. Meyer adopted the following consensus: in the absence of a response to corticosteroid therapy, second-line treatment should be started rapidly, without attempting to prolong or increase corticosteroid therapy, by proposing either splenectomy or the use of rituximab [23].

An observation made in a sickle-cell, thalassemic, polytransfused patient shows the favorable action of rituximab on both AACs and allo-ACs. This observation is an example of the value of rituximab in dramatic transfusion situations [23].

4.5.1.4. Immunosuppressants

None of our patients received immunosuppressive therapy.

Indeed, because of the potential risks to patients, immunosuppressive therapy should be considered primarily in cases of AHAI refractory to corticosteroid therapy, splenectomy and rituximab, or for those resistant to these medical treatments and unsuitable for surgery [14, 17]. The most commonly used therapeutic agents are azathioprine and ciclosporin, 6-mercaptopurine and cytotoxic agents such as vincristine and cyclophosphamide. Overall, the response rate varies from 40% to 60% [2, 84].

4.5.1.5.   Intravenous immunoglobulin (IVIG)

IVIg was administered to 3 patients in our series (17.6%). No remarkable effects were observed.

High-dose intravenous immunoglobulins (2-5 g/kg/d) have been the subject of only isolated reports or small open-label studies [13, 14, 22]. They are not a recommended first-line treatment for isolated AHAI. This treatment can be used in severe, cortico-resistant forms. Success is inconsistent but real [6, 12].

4.5.1.6.   Transfusion therapy

In our series, almost all patients (16/17) received blood transfusions, 4 of whom were beta thalassemic and therefore transfusion-dependent. Transfusion performance was good in 4/16 cases and moderate in 8/16 patients.

The indication for transfusion is not based solely on the hemoglobin level, but rather on the clinical tolerance of the anemia. Patients with chronic anemia are in most cases asymptomatic and do not generally require transfusion. Transfusions are therefore indicated in cases of severe anemia [2, 17].

In the series by Habibi .B et al. the number of patients with acute AHAI was 34/80 (42.5%). Of these, some 67.6% (23/34) required blood transfusions, which were effective in only 5/23 patients. None of the chronic AHAIs required blood transfusions [41].

The general rule is therefore to avoid blood transfusions whenever possible, because of their transient effects and, above all, their immunological risks [17].

In AHAI, transfusion therapy comes up against several problems:

- The limited lifespan of transfused red blood cells.
- The difficulty with cross-matching is finding compatible blood: most AACs react with all potential blood donors.
- The coexistence in the patient's serum of an allo-AC that may be masked by the AAC [2, 17].

Under these conditions, the search for the "least incompatible" blood bags is not generally useful. Rather, two other procedures arise: if the patient has never been transfused, the transfused RBCs and his own RBCs have the same survival in the presence of AACs, and the risk of having associated allo-ACs is very rare, so the patient can be transfused even with incompatible bags. On the other hand, if the child has already undergone previous transfusions, the coexistence of allo-AC and AAC is very likely. The adsorption technique is therefore needed to identify the associated allo-AC and transfuse phenotyped RBC concentrates [2].

4.5.1.7.   Folic acid

In our series, only 2 patients (11.8%) benefited from folate supplementation. This treatment is designed to compensate for the vitamin deficiency caused by high bone marrow regenerative activity (accelerated erythropoiesis) [1].

4.5.1.8.   Other therapeutic means

Plasma exchange in a heated extracorporeal circuit may be proposed for certain chronic cold agglutinin carriers who are clinically handicapped and refractory to simpler treatments [6]. This therapy has been used successfully, but its indication seems reserved for severe AHAI uncontrolled by other means [14]. However, some authors have shown that this method has only limited effects over time, and is unlikely to lead to a sustained clinical response [4, 35].

Experience with hematopoietic stem cell transplantation in refractory immune cytopenias was recently summarized by Pession et al, who concluded that transplantation can be effective in around half of cases, but with a high mortality rate (26%) [85].

The efficacy of danazol, an androgen with weak androgenic action, has also been proven in the treatment of IgG + complement and complement-type AHAI [14].

4.5.2. Special case of "hot" IgM AHAI

IgM hot AHAI is generally refractory to conventional therapies effective in IgG hot AHAI including steroids, IVIG, and splenectomy. Some studies have shown the efficacy of rituximab, interferon alpha 2b, eculizumab and bortezomib in the treatment of this form of AHAI [35].

The use of rituximab in combination with eculizumab further improved the course of the disease, leading to complete normalization of the clinico-biological signs of hemolysis [86].

4.5.3. Treatment of "cold" AHAI

Only one case of "cold" AHAI (HBDL) was suspected in our patients.

The literature shows that the management of "cold" HAIs is indeed radically different from that of "hot" HAIs. Some AHAIs, particularly those that are clearly post-infectious, can heal spontaneously [12]. Therapeutic management of FAD is usually limited to purely symptomatic measures to prevent cold [26]. Good hydration and diuresis are also important to avoid the toxic effects of hemoglobinuria on the renal tubules [2]. In 50% of cases, anemia is moderate and requires no drug treatment [87]. Corticosteroid therapy and splenectomy (hemolysis being intrahepatic) are notoriously ineffective, and immunosuppressive drugs are highly inconsistent in preventing hemolysis flares [26].

In symptomatic and severe forms, rituximab offers an attractive therapeutic alternative. The initial results of treatment with this agent are very promising, with a response of around 50-60%. In addition, this drug can be used in cases of renal failure, but some authors suggest that these responses are generally relatively short-lived [22, 26, 87].

The combination of rituximab and fludarabine has further improved the prognostic outcome in AFM, with an overall response rate of 75% [19, 88]. Compared with fludarabine, bendamustine has few adverse effects and excellent clinical tolerability. Thus, the combination of bendamustine with rituximab could be an effective chemoimmunotherapy, especially in the elderly. Gueli.A et al. have demonstrated the importance of this combination in the treatment of MAF and, in general, in AHAI associated with non-Hodgkin's lymphoma [19].

4.5.4. Treatment of drug-induced AHAI

In our series, we have a single case of AHAI probably secondary to ibuprofen and/or augmentin, with TCD negativation and disappearance of signs of hemolysis simply by discontinuing treatment in the absence of any other therapy.

According to the literature, the essential step is, of course, definitive discontinuation of the drug. The classic therapeutic means envisaged for classic AHAI can be used. Plasma exchange, which has been used in this context to eliminate the drug and/or its metabolites from the circulation [14, 89], has a special place.

4.6. Evolution

4.6.1. Prognostic factors

In our study, 62.5% of IgG+C3d TCD AHAIs had progressed to chronicity. Moreover, 5/8 (62.5%) of patients with chronic AHAI were under 4 years of age.

In children, three prognostic factors, present from the initial diagnosis onwards, suggest an unfavorable evolution and the need for rigorous specialized monitoring: age under 4 years, abnormal immunoglobulin weight assay and IgG/IgG+C3d type CDT. According to the literature, there is a greater risk of chronic evolution if the CDT is IgG or mixed in childhood AHAI [28, 39].

4.6.2. Evolving forms

With the exception of a single patient whose AHAI course was not specified, in our study we distinguished between an acute form (8/17) and a chronic form (8/17). According to other series, the frequency of occurrence of these forms varies from 25% to 77% [39, 41].

Acute AHAI evolved significantly towards complete recovery and cure in 75% of cases (P= 0.018). Our results are in line with the literature, since the evolution of acute forms is generally favorable, and cure is reflected by disappearance of the anemia and negativation of the TCD [22, 39].

4.6.3. Mortality

In our series, 9/17 patients (52.9%) were cured, while 2 died. Both of these cases followed acute post-infectious (leishmaniasis) AHAI of abrupt onset. Older series of childhood HAIs reported a high mortality rate (11-32%) in chronic HAIs [12]. In adults, the mortality rate is higher (28-70%). In fact, this difference could be due to the predominance of transient acute forms, the rarity of malignancies associated with AHAI, and probably to the good sensitivity of children to the various therapeutic agents [41].

In 2014,Vagace and colleagues showed that, in children, mortality from AHAI generally due to infection, hemolysis or underlying disease, has decreased over the years from around 30% to less than 5% [2]. The regression in mortality rates over the years correlates well with advances in knowledge of this pathology, especially in clinical-biological and therapeutic terms.

4.6.4. Complications

In our series, we noted two types of complications: cardiac damage linked to AHAI itself, and signs of cortisone impregnation linked to prolonged corticosteroid therapy.

In addition, it has been reported that the duration and cumulative doses of corticosteroids expose the majority of patients to numerous adverse effects, and in particular to an increased risk of infections. Other possible complications of AHAI include an increased risk of deep vein thrombosis. This risk appears to be particularly high in patients with antiphospholipid AC and/or a history of splenectomy [22].

Conclusion

Although the pathophysiology and diagnosis of AHAIs are now better understood, they remain a complex and heterogeneous group of pathologies. The exact mechanism of AHAI, whether idiopathic or disease-associated, remains a matter of theoretical debate. But the pathophysiology of hemolysis is currently well understood, and the correlation between classical serological data and clinical pictures remains relevant.

The diagnosis of AHAI relies on a simple but rigorous interpretation of immunohematological parameters, and a number of complementary tests are also necessary to avoid overlooking associated pathology.

In more complex cases (e.g. lack of initial orientation, poly-pathological and/or polytransfused patients), more specific tests may be required. In such cases, collaboration between clinicians and biologists is even more important, in order to assess the relevance and/or expected cost-effectiveness of the various tests on a case-by-case basis, and to ensure that results are correctly interpreted, particularly in the case of recently transfused patients. Anti-erythrocyte immunization represents a serious problem in patients with hemoglobinopathies and therefore polytransfused, especially given the increase in transfusion indications in the management of these patients. This calls for a preventive transfusion strategy to ensure optimal safety and vigilance in monitoring transfusion therapy.

At present, even if new approaches appear promising both now and in the future, the management of AHAI remains a function of the severity of the anemia and sensitivity to the various treatments used. The use of these different treatments remains essentially based on the experience of the clinicians who manage these patients.

The emergence of new therapies such as rituximab should enable us to broaden treatment regimens and, initially, improve treatment of forms of AHAI that are inaccessible to conventional therapies.

Bibliography

1. Michel M. Warm autoimmune hemolytic anemia: Advances in pathophysiology and treatment. Presse Med. 2014; 43: 97-104.

2. Vagace JM , Bajo R , Gervasini G. Diagnostic and therapeutic challenges of primary autoimmune haemolytic anaemia in children. Arch Dis Child. 2014; 99: 668-673.

3. Mack P, Freedman J. Autoimmune Hemolytic Anemia: A History. Transfus Med Rev. 2000; 14: 223-233.

4. Grattay G. Immune hemolytic anemia caused by drugs. Expert Opin Drug Saf. 2012; 11: 635-642.

5. Bonnotte B. Pathogenic mechanism of autoimmune disease. Rev Med Interne. 2004; 25: 648-658.

6. Habibi B. Autoimmune hemolytic anemias. Sem ther hop. 1989; 65: 1465-1477.

7. Guitton C, Ledeist F, Tchernia G, Bader-meunier B. Autoimmune hemolytic anemia and dyserythropoiesis revealing a Fas apoptosis deficiency in 3 children. Arch Pediatr. 2006; 13: 367-370.

8. Hall AM, Ward FJ, Vickers MA, Stott LM, Urbaniak SJ, Barker RN. Interleukin-10 mediated regulatory T-cell responses to epitopes on a human red blood cell autoantigen. Blood. 2002; 100: 4529-4536.

9. Ahmad E, Elgohari T, Ibrahim H. Naturally occurring regulatory T cells and interleukins 10 and 12 in the pathogenesis of idiopathic warm autoimmune hemolytic anemia. J Investig Allergol Clin Immunol. 2011; 21: 297-304.

10. Bass GF, Tuscano ET, Tuscano JM. Diagnosis and classification of autoimmune hemolytic anemia. Autoimmun Rev. 2014; 1486: 1-5.

11. Jarrassé C, Pagnier A, Edan C, Landman-Parker J, Mazingued F, Mansuy L et al. Hodgkin's disease and autoimmunity in children: about 11 observations. Arch Pediatr. 2011; 18: 376-382.

12. Aladjidi N, Leverger G, Pariente A, Bader-Meunier B, Le Deist F, Colin Y et al. Epidemiology of autoimmune haemolytic anemia in children: French data. Arch Pediatr. 2006; 13: 511-521.

13. Philippe P. Diagnosis and management of autoimmune hemolytic anemia. Presse Med. 2007; 36: 1959-1969.

14. Le Pennec PY, Rouger P. Immunologic hemolytic anemias: From autoimmunity to anti-drug immunization. Transfus Clin Biol. 1995; 2: 123-133.

15. Zeerleder S. Autoimmune hemolytic anemia - a diagnostic and therapeutic challenge. Forum Med Suisse. 2010; 10: 626-633.

16. Berentsen S, Beiske K, Tjonnfjord GE. Primary chronic cold agglutinin disease: an update on pathogenesis, clinical features and therapy. Hematol. 2007; 12: 361-370.

17. Packman CH. Hemolytic anemia due to warm autoantibodies. Blood Rev. 2008; 22: 17-31.

18. Lambert JF, Nydegger UE. Geoepidemiology of autoimmune hemolytic anemia. Autoimmu Rev. 2010; 9: 350-354.

19. Gueli A, Gottardi D, Hu H, Ricca I, De Crescenzo A, Tarella C. Efficacy

of rituximab-bendamustine in cold agglutinin haemolytic anaemia refractory to previous chemo-immunotherapy: a case report. Blood Transfus. 2013; 11: 311-314.

20. Grimaldi D, Limal N, Noizat-Pirenne F, Janvier D, Godeau B, Michel M. Coombs IgA autoimmune hemolytic anemia revealing hepatitis C virus infection. Rev Med Interne. 2008; 29: 135-138.

21. Bernard C, Bollotte A, Bricca P , Vial T, Broussolle C, Sève P. Les anémies hémolytiques immunologiques médicamenteuses : étude rétrospective de 10 observations. Rev Med Interne. 2014; 4785: 1-11.

22. Michel M. Characteristics of "hot" antibody autoimmune hemolytic anemias and Evans syndrome in adults. Presse Med. 2008; 37: 1309-1318.

23. Rigal D, Meyer F. Autoimmune hemolytic anemias: biological diagnosis and new therapeutic approaches. Transfus Clin Biol. 2011; 18: 277-285.

24. Palla AR, Khimani F, Craig MD. Warm Autoimmune Hemolytic Anemia with a Direct Antiglobulin Test Positive for C3 and Negative for IgG: A case Study and Analytical Literature Review of Incidence and Severity. Clin Med Insights Case Rep. 2013; 6: 57-60.

25. Moncharmont P, Sanchez C, Dijoux L, Neyraval N, Rigal D. Prevalence of IgA antired blood cell autoantibodies as observed through direct antiglobulin test. Immunol Anal Biol Spec. 2008; 23: 58-60.

26. SekkachY , Hammi S , Elqatni M, Fatihi J , Elomri N, Mekouar Fet al. Exemplary efficacy of rituximab in a case of cold autoantibody hemolytic anemia. Ann Pharm Fr. 2011; 69: 205-208.

27. Valentine L, Constance G, Garcon L , Bertrand G, Michel M. Hemolytic anemia in adults: main causes and diagnostic approach. Presse Med. 2011; 40: 470-485.

28. Leverger C, Fischer A, Revillon Y, Griscelli C. Autoimmune hemolytic anemia in children. 14 case reports. Arch Fr Pediatr. 1984; 41: 665-671.

29. Genty I, Michel M, Hermine O, Schaeffer A, Godeau B, Rochant H. Characteristics of autoimmune hemolytic anemias in adults: retrospective analysis of a series of 83 patients. Rev Med Interne. 2002; 23: 901-909.

30. Nathalie A, Guy L, Leblanc T, Picat MQ, Michel G, Bertrand Y et al. New insights into childhood autoimmune hemolytic anemia: a French national observational study of 265 children. Haematol. 2011; 96: 655-663.

31. Giovannetti G, Pauselli S, Barrella G, Neri A, Antonetti L, Gentile G et al. Severe warm autoimmune haemolytic anaemia due to anti-Jka autoantibody associated with Parvovirus B19 infection in a child. Blood Transfus. 2013; 11: 634-635.

32. Bercovitz RS, Macy M, Ambruso DR. A case of autoimmune hemolytic anemia with anti-D specificity in one-year-old. Immunohematology. 2013; 29: 15-18.

33. Eddou H, Helissey C, Konopacki J, Souleau B, de Revel T, Malfuson JV. Evans syndrome: beware of overdiagnosis. Rev Med Interne. 2012; 33: 155-158.

34. Segel GB, Lichtman MA. Direct antiglobulin ("Coombs") test-negative

autoimmune hemolytic anemia: A review. Blood Cells Mol Dis. 2013; 16: 19.

35. Chao MP, Hong J, Kunder C, Lester L, Schrier SL, Majeti R. Refractory warm IgM-mediated autoimmune hemolytic anemia associated with Churg- Strauss syndrome responsive to eculizumab and rituximab. Am J Hematol. 2014; 45: 1-4.

36. Oytip N, Sriwanitchrak P, Tubrod J, Kupatawintu P. Antibody elutions in Thai patients with a positive direct antiglobulin test. Blood Transfus. 2011; 9: 306-310.

37. Kumar KJ, Kumar HCK, Manjunath VJ, Arun V. Autoimmune Hemolytic Anemia due to Varicella Infection. Iran J Pediatr. 2013; 23: 491-492.

38. Vaglio S, Arista MC, Perrone MP, Tomei G, Testi AM, Coluzzi S. Autoimmune hemolytic anemia in childhood: serologic features in 100 cases. Transfusion. 2007; 47: 50-54.

39. Jezequel Ch, Le Gall E, Patillon S, Guerin MN. Autoimmune hemolytic anemias in children about 14 observations. Rev Pediatr. 1986;125: 51-58.

40. Tantawy AAG, Al-Tawil MM. Spectrum and outcome of autoimmune hemolytic anemia in children: single-center experience in 10 years. Eg J Haematol. 2014; 39: 20-24.

41. Habibi B, Homberg JC, Schaison G, Salmon C. Autoimmune Hemolytic Anemia in Children: A Review of 80 Cases. Am J Med. 1974; 56: 61-69.

42. McGann PT, McDade J, Mortier NA, Combs MR, Ware RE. IgA-Mediated Autoimmune Hemolytic Anemia in an Infant. Pediatr Blood Cancer. 2011; 56: 837-839.

43. Sokol RJ, Hewitt S, Stamps BK, Hitchen PA. Autoimmune Haemolysis in Childhood and Adolescence. Acta haematol. 1984; 72: 245-257.

44. Goudemand M, Salmon C. Autoimmune hemolytic anemias. In: Immuno-hématologie et immunogénétique. Paris: Flammarion; 1980: 393411.

45. Oucheri M, Chakroun T, Abdelkefi S , Houissa B, Romdhane H, Jemni Yaacoub S. Anti D autoimmunization in a patient with weak D type 4.0. Transfus Clin Biol. 2013; 15: 1-4.

46. Kaneko S, Sato M, Sasaki G, Eguchi H, Oishi T, Kamesaki T et al. Case of cytomegalovirus-associated direct anti-globulin test-negative autoimmune hemolytic anemia. Pediatr Int. 2013; 43: 785-788.

47. Shizuma T. A Patient with Alcoholic Liver Cirrhosis Who Developed Autoimmune Hemolytic Anemia Following Infection with Influenza Type A. JSM Biotechnol Bioeng. 2014; 2:1-3.

48. Chen H, Jia XL, Gao HM, Qian SY. Comorbid presentation of severe novel influenza A (H1N1) and Evans syndrome: a case report. Chin Med J. 2011; 124: 1743-1746.

49. Schoindre Y, Bollée G, Dumont MD , Lesavre P, Servais A. Cold agglutinin syndrome associated with a 2009 influenza A H1N1 infection. Am J Med. 2011; 124: 1-2.

50. Gruson B, Veyssier P, Coquin-Radeau E, Juszczak M, Darnige L.

Autoimmune hemolytic anemia caused by IgG cold agglutinins after infectous mononucleosis. Rev Med Interne. 2004; 25: 764-772.

51. Calvaruso V, Craxi A. Immunological alterations in hepatitis C virus infection. World J Gastroenterol. 2013; 19: 8916-8923.

52. Thapa R, Ghosh A. Childhood autoimmune hemolytic anemia following hepatitis E virus infection. J Paediatr Child Health. 2009; 45: 71-72.

53. Rafalli J, Harmouche H, Benjilali L, Tazi-Mezalek Z, Adnaoui M, Aouini M et al. Autoimmune hemolytic anemia: An unusual revelation of human immunodeficiency virus. Presse Med. 2010; 39: 840-842.

54. Edmar A, Piyarali S, Boumahni B, Bangui A, Renouil M. Autoimmune hemolytic anemia and Mycoplasma pneumoniae pneumopathy. Arch Pediatr. 1997; 4: 1016-1022.

55. Erduran E, Bahadir A, Gedik Y. Kala-Azar associated withCoombs-positive autoimmune hemolytic anemia in the patients coming from the andemic area of the disease and successful treatement of these patients with liposomal amphotericin B. Pediatr Hematol Oncol. 2005; 22: 349-355.

56. Mahajan V, Marwaha RK. Immune Mediated Hemolysis in Visceral Leishmaniasis. J Trop Pediatr. 2007; 53: 284-286.

57. Braham D, Klii R, Bouteraa W, Harzllah O, Graja S, Mahjoub S. Visceral leishmaniasis associated with warm autoantibody hemolytic anemia. Rev Med Interne. 2008; 29: 380-381.

58. Nozzi M, Del Torto M, Chiarelli F, Breda L. Leishmaniasis and

autoimmune diseases in pediatric age. Cell Immunol. 2014; 292: 9-13.

59. Teulade J, Gay C, Rabeyrin H. A diagnostic dilemma: visceral leishmaniasis with hyperglobulinemia and positive Coombs test masquerading as an auto immune hepatitis in a three-year-old girl. Rev Med Interne. 2008; 29: 85-88.

60. Zuckerman A. Current Status of the Immunology of Malaria and of the Antigenic Analysis of Plasmodia A Five-Year Review. Bull Wld Hlth Org. 1969; 40: 55-56.

61. Singh D, Gupta V, Acharya S, Mahajan SN, Verma A. A case of plasmodium vivax malaria associated with severe autoimmune hemolytic anaemia. Ann Trop Med Public Health. 2012; 5: 133-136.

62. Johnson AS, Delisca G, Booth GS. Warm autoimmune hemolytic anemia secondary to Plasmodium ovale infection: A case report and review of the literature. Transfus Apheresis Sci. 2013; 49: 571-573.

63. Delphine G, Busse JB, Cunningham-Rundles C, Galicier L, Dechartres A,
Berezne A et al. Efficacy and safety of rituximab in common variable immunodeficiency-associated immune cytopenias: a retrospective multicentre study on 33 patients. Br J Haematol. 2011; 155: 498-508.

64. Park CY, Chung CH. A Patient with Mixed Type Evans Syndrome: Efficacy of Rituximab Treatment. J Korean Med Sci. 2006; 21: 1115-1116.

65. Sève P, Broussolle C, Pavic M. Primary immune deficiencies and autoimmune cytopenias in adults. Rev Med Interne. 2013; 34:148-153.

66. Ben Amor I, Louati N, Khemekhem H, Dhieb A, Rekik H, Mdhaffar M et al. Anti-erythrocyte immunization in hemoglobinopathies: about 84 cases. Transfus Clin Biol. 2012; 19: 345-352.

67. Guirat-Dhouib N, Mezri M, Hmida H, Mellouli F, Kaabi H, Ouderni M et al.. High frequency of autoimmunization among transfusion-dependent Tunisian thalassaemia patients. Transfus Apher Sci. 2011; 45:199-202.

68. Kim I, Lee JY, Kwon JH, Jung JY, Song HH, Park Yl et al. A Case of Autoimmune Hemolytic Anemia Associated with an Ovarian Teratoma. J Korean Med Sci. 2006; 21: 365-367.

69. Guillaume N, Alimardani G, Chatelain D, Henry X, Claisse JF. Disappearance of autoantibodies inducing hemolysis after resection of gastric stromal tumor Description of a case and review of the literature. Rev Med Interne. 2003; 24: 131-135.

70. Glorieux I, Chabbert V, Rubie H, Baunin C, Gaspard M, Guitard J et al. Autoimmune hemolytic anemia associated with mature teratoma of the ovary. Arch Pediatr. 1998; 5: 41-44.

71. Grigoriadis C, Tympa A, Liapis A, Hassiakos D, Bakas P. AlphaMethyldopa-Induced Autoimmune Hemolytic Anemia in the Third Trimester of Pregnancy. Case Rep Obstet Gynecol. 2013; 2013: 1-2.

72. Salmeron G, Molina TJ, Fieschi C, Zagdanski AM, Brice P, Sibon D. Autoimmune Hemolytic Anemia and Nodular Lymphocyte-Predominant Hodgkin Lymphoma: A Rare Association. Case Rep

Hematol. 2013; 2013: 1-5.

73. D'Arena G, Guariglia R, La Rocca F, Trino S, Condelli V, De Martino L et al. Autoimmune Cytopenias in Chronic Lymphocytic Leukemia. Clin Dev Immunol. 2013; 2013: 1-8.

74. Moreno C, Hodgson K, Ferrer G, Elena M, Filella X, Pereira A et al. Autoimmune cytopenia in chronic lymphocytic leukemia: prevalence, clinical associations, and prognostic significance. Blood. 2010; 116: 47714776.

75. Zent CS, Kay NE. Autoimmune Complications in Chronic Lymphocytic. Best Pract Res Clin Haemato. 2010; 23: 47-59.

76. Barbaryan A, Iyinagoro C, Nwankwo N, Ali AM, Saba R, Kwatra SG et al. Ibuprofen-Induced Hemolytic Anemia. Case Rep Hematol. 2013; 2013:1-3.

77. Garratty G , Arndt PA. An update on drug-induced immune haemolytic anemia. Immunohematol. 2007; 23: 105-119.

78. Bardon J, Mirault T, Hessaine S, Minozzi C, Rappoport M, Messas E et al. Rifampicin, an exceptional cause of drug-induced hemolytic anemia. Rev Med Interne. 2010; 31: 479-480.

79. David S. Anemia and medications. Rev fr allergol. 2009; 49: 44-48.

80. Chauffrey L, Chamouni P, Bégarina L, Benhamoua Y, Cailleuxa N, Borg JY et al. MYH9 syndrome and autoimmune hemolytic anemia: a chance association. Rev Med Interne. 2012; 33: 99-102.

81. Giulino LB, Bussel JB, Neufeld EJ. Treatment with rituximab in benign

and malignant hematologic disorders in children. J Pediatr. 2007; 150: 338-344.

82. Stasi R. Rituximab in autoimmune hematologic diseases: not just a matter of B cells. Semin Hematol. 2010; 47: 170-179.

83. Penalver FJ, Alvarez-Larran A, Diez-Martin JL, Gallur L, Jarque I, Caballero D et al. Rituximab is an effective and safe therapeutic alternative in adults with refractory and severe autoimmune hemolytic anemia. Ann Hematol. 2010; 89: 1073-1080.

84. Sobota A, Neufeld EJ, Lapsia S, Bennett CM. Response to mercaptopurine for refractory autoimmune cytopenias in children. Pediatr Blood Cancer. 2009; 52: 80-84.

85. Pession A, Zama D, Masetti R, Gasperini P, Prete A. Hematopoietic stem cell transplantation for curing children with severe autoimmune diseases: is this a valid option. Pediatr Transplant. 2012; 16: 413-425.

86. Swiecicki PL, Hegerova LT, Gertz MA. Cold agglutinin disease. Blood. 2013; 122: 1114-1121.

87. Palombi M, Niscola P, Trawinska MM, Scaramucci L, Giovannini M, Perrotti A et al. Long-lasting remission induced by rituximab in two cases of refractory autoimmune haemolytic anaemia due to cold agglutinins. Blood Transfus. 2009; 7: 235-236.

88. Berentsen S. Therapy for chronic cold agglutinin disease: perspective for further improvements. Blood Transfus. 2013; 11: 167-168.

89. Garratty G. Immune haemolytic anemia associated with drug therapy.

Blood Rev. 2010; 24: 143-150.